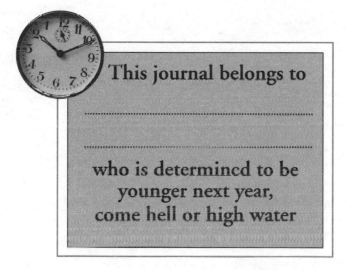

This journal belongs to

....

....

who is determined to be
younger next year,
come hell or high water

Based on *The New York Times* bestseller

Younger Next Year Journal

You're serious about exercise and eating better. Now it's time to write things down. It could make all the difference.

Chris Crowley &
Henry S. Lodge, M.D.

Workman Publishing · New York

Library of Congress Cataloging-in-Publication Data is available.

ISBN 978-0-7611-4469-4

Workman books are available at special discounts when purchased in
bulk for premiums and sales promotions as well as for fund-raising or
educational use. Special editions or book excerpts can also be created
to specification. For details, contact the Special Sales Director at the
address below, or send an e-mail to specialmarkets@workman.com

Workman Publishing Company, Inc.
225 Varick Street
New York, NY 10014-4381
www.workman.com
www.youngernextyear.com

Printed in the United States of America
Perfect-bound edition first printing October 2011

10 9 8 7 6 5 4

Nice Going!

Everyone *says* they want to be Younger Next Year. But you, you decent creature, are actually *doing* something about it. You have taken the critical first step. You have spent hard cash money for this journal, and there is at least a *chance* that you will use it. Excellent. Because that is the single best thing you can do to motivate yourself over time to do all the stuff that Harry (that will be Dr. Henry S. Lodge, M.D., the coauthor of the *Younger Next Year* books and my close pal) and I promise is the key to living like a much younger man or woman well into your eighties and beyond. Stuff like doing serious exercise six days a week, and giving up the lunatic national pastime of eating mountains of crap every day, and acting like the mammal you are by staying in meaningful touch with your fellow creatures. Keep this journal and you will do that stuff. Do that stuff and you will get Younger Next Year.

Dr. Harry Lodge (left) has come up with a plan for turning back your biological clock; Chris Crowley is proof that it works.

WHAT'S IN IT FOR YOU? PLENTY!

By the way, we realize that keeping this journal isn't going to make perfect sense unless you've taken a peek at one of the *Younger Next Year* books. But in case you haven't read them—and because we're so eager to get you into this essential business of journal-keeping—here's a quick summary of where we're coming from . . . and where we hope you're going.

The core premise of the books is that there is a major revolution in aging at hand. Follow seven simple rules—and keep track of how well you follow them in this journal—and you can avoid up to 70 percent of normal, American aging, as well as up to 50 percent of all the serious sickness and accidents that afflict most people from the time they're fifty until the day they die. Aging, it turns out, is voluntary. Don't volunteer!

So, here are the rules as outlined by Harry. They're simple. Thing is, you have to follow them for the rest of your life. But the payoff is huge, so pay attention.

HARRY'S RULES

- **Exercise six days a week for the rest of your life.**
- **Do serious aerobic exercise four days a week for the rest of your life.**
- **Do serious strength training, with weights, two days a week for the rest of your life.**
- **Spend less than you make.**
- **Quit eating crap!**
- **Care.**
- **Connect and commit.**

These rules may seem a little extreme. Okay, very extreme, some of them. But when you think of the payoff—avoiding up to

70 percent of usual aging—they are a walk on the beach. A rather long and difficult walk, perhaps, but well worth it. Still, you need to motivate yourself—in the beginning and for the long haul. And the single best thing for that is to keep a journal.

Keeping a journal has *really* worked for me. (Sorry, don't mean to confuse you—this is Chris talking now.) I have carried a log of my own devising everywhere I go for years. And I have written down (in more or less detail) all the exercise I did, and a lot of what I ate. Or drank. Some days it's fun because I've been a good guy. And some days it's a litany of shame. But every stinking day, no matter what, I write the stuff down—good, bad, or ugly. And it helps more than any other single thing to keep me motivated . . . to keep me at it.

From time to time, I have lost the book; *immediately,* I have gone to hell. It is uncanny: If there is no record, it's as if no one cares. And if no one cares . . . well, you're down the rat hole in a second. Believe me, forget the journal and it's as if the teacher has left the room and we can all be bad. Which is absurd—after all, no one but me will ever see the thing. Who cares?

I do. In some weird way, keeping the journal is my way of saying, "I care. And I am keeping track. So let's be serious here." It is a little covenant with myself, a matter of taking myself seriously, which is always a tricky business. It is an indispensable key to actually doing some of the stuff I promise myself to do. Like getting out of bed and going to the gym or out on the bike almost every day of my life. Or resisting the deep-seated desire to eat a package of Oreos. Knowing that I have to write it down makes a surprising difference. It radically improves my chances of being a semi-decent human being.

So give it a shot and see if keeping a journal works for you. Make yourself use it for a week. See what happens. Oh, and start today. Don't wait for something big. This is a humble little book, and it's okay to start small. Just make some entry every day. It may make all the difference. It's just like the business of doing exercise itself: There will be days when you don't feel like it or you just can't. But do some damn thing anyway, no matter how modest. And write it down, no matter how puny. Write something every single day. It'll keep you going. It matters.

THE DREARY BUT NECESSARY BUSINESS OF SETTING GOALS

I have looked at a bunch of journals like this over the years and have never gotten much beyond the first page. The authors always begin by telling me about how I should be "setting goals" for my life. Which makes me cranky . . . probably because their ideas and mine are so different. Most of them want me to think about "improving my time" in this or that race. And the whole thing seems to be about setting cycles—ramping up what I'm doing in a series of steps—so I'll be ready for that big event. Except I'm not going to enter a race anytime soon, and I bet you're not either. So, the hell with it, and the hell with slowly and agonizingly building up for this and that. It all looks like Lance Armstrong country to me, and I'm not going.

What I want—and what may be a help to you, too—is a simple journal that will help me exercise hard enough and steadily enough for the rest of my life to feel good, so that I can do things and have fun. (And *be* fun, come to think of it.) In my experience—and I've been at this for quite a few years now—just fitting that amount of exercise into a day takes a whole lot of work and some pretty serious motivation.

Which is why I have slowly and reluctantly come to the conclusion that setting goals really does help. And why I risk turning you all off by actually suggesting that you take a half hour or so and think of some things you'd like to do over the next year or two . . . some places you'd like to go. You don't have to drive yourself nuts over this; goals can be intensely personal and idiosyncratic, like swimming around that little island on the lake you go to by next August first. Or doing a fifty-mile bike ride by next September . . . in under five hours. Whatever. August first. Next September. You decide. What Harry and I are going to do is mention some of the goals that we have set for ourselves in recent times. They may give you some ideas. Then again, they may not.

CHRIS'S GOALS

Okeydoke, here we go. But remember, I am a reasonably fit 72-year-old guy who's been doing this for a while. My goals will look namby-pamby to some of you and appallingly ambitious to others. Don't worry about it . . . they're just food for thought. Something to get *you* thinking about *your* life in this Next Third that Harry and I say can be so terrific. You know, like you really can be a functional fifty-year-old at seventy . . . feel it and act it in all the important ways, if you get off your butt and move.

Biking: I bike like crazy, but I'm oddly slow for the amount of time I spend at it. So, here are some little goals: First, I'd like to get so I'm doing my regular, sixteen-mile loop (lots of hills) in an hour and ten minutes. For me, that's wildly ambitious. Second, I'd like to do a fifty-mile spin—again, up in the hills near my place—at an average speed of 13 miles an hour. That's a lot slower than many men in their forties, fifties, and sixties would be aiming for, but it would be a major push for me. Third, I am going biking in Ireland with some pals in six months; I'd like to be in good enough shape to ride, at least part of the time, with the "A" group. And I want to go on that "century" bike ride that Harry's going to tell you about soon.

Single Sculling: I also like to row a lot. It's a sport almost no one does, but it's super exercise that often takes you through beautiful settings. My goal here is a surprise even to me. I actually *do* want to enter a race . . . Boston's Head of the Charles in October. I did it once before (the second race I'd entered in fifty years) and I aspire to improve my time by a minute. (I'd be satisfied to finish, to tell the truth; writing down this "goal" will at least force me to enroll.)

Weights: I would like to be able to leg-press 500 pounds (three sets of ten) by the beginning of next ski season . . . say December 31. That's a hell of a lot, but my legs are pretty good. And I'd love to be able to bicep-curl 50 pounds (three sets of ten) and do 100 sit-ups. That's not much, but my core strength isn't great, so it's plenty good enough.

Being There: But my most important and most serious goal is just to *be there*, six days a week, fifty-two weeks a year—four days of serious aerobics (with some interval work) and two or three days of weights . . . each week.

Weight Loss: This is just what we tell you not to do in the books. Our advice is not to try to diet at all because 95 percent of all diets fail. Just "quit eating crap" and exercise six days a week; the weight loss will come over time. We stick by this superb advice. But I'm desperate to drop a few pounds. I'm going to give it a shot and promise myself not to get mopey if it doesn't work . . . it's a minor part of fitness and youth. So, here goes: I would like to weigh 170 by my next birthday and 165 by the next Head of the Charles sculling race, come October. My weight's been creeping up again and I want to turn it around. I am not talking about a diet . . . just cranking up the lifestyle a bit. Doing a little more exercise, and eating just a hair less crap.

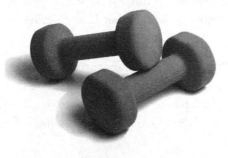

HARRY'S GOALS

 More Weights: Surprisingly enough, even after writing the books, I have fallen off track a little with the weights. I have stuck with six days a week of exercise, but I have been doing almost entirely aerobic work, and I feel it. Mostly in my shoulders, but I am aware that my knees and ankles are next on the list. My goal is to hit strength training two to three days a week for a couple or three months and then back off to twice a week. I plan to use mostly light weights at higher repetitions over the first three months, since I find it perilously easy to overdo it.

Ride a Century: I've just bought a new bike, after twenty-six years on the old one, and I want to work up to riding a century (100 miles). I'm not going to set a time frame for that, because in my case it depends on tendons more than muscles. Still, I want to get there within six months or so, if not sooner. For me, just having that goal on paper is enough to start pulling me out the door for longer rides.

Have the Right Food Available: I've pretty much quit eating crap, but I'm not perfect by any stretch, so I'm going to focus on building more fruits and vegetables into my daily routine. I find that a lot of good nutrition is simply planning to have the right food around, and then eating it. In most people's lives, the wrong food is always around, and often it's the easiest to go with. My goal for this next year is simply to be sure the right food is as easy to get to as the wrong food!

NOW IT'S YOUR TURN

Depending on where you are in your life, your goals may resemble ours, or you may decide—totally correctly and with real commitment—to aim for something much smaller. For you, a five-mile walk around your local park might be a real achievement.

If so, go for it! On the other hand, if you're in pretty good shape, you may want to try for something beyond our imaginations. Godspeed. But whatever your goals, it's now your turn to write them down.

MY GOALS

1. _____

_____

_____

2. _____

_____

_____

3. _____

_____

_____

4. _____

_____

_____

5. _____

_____

_____

6. _____

_____

_____

7. _____

_____

_____

GET A HEART RATE MONITOR

We are nuts on this subject, but only because it makes your workouts so much more interesting and effective. We know you hate the idea, but go get a heart rate monitor and put it on. It'll keep you honest and motivated. We both use Polar brand heart monitors, and the cheapest ones (which cost around fifty bucks) are just as useful for the average person as the more expensive ones. You can find them at any local sports store. What you get doesn't much matter. You just need something that will measure your heart rate in beats per minute, because that is the simplest, most reliable way to tell how hard you are working out.

A heart monitor will also allow you to track your aerobic workouts in terms of "percent of maximum heart rate." And that's what we want you to do. "Percent of maximum heart rate? Huh?" Now is the point at which 64 percent of you are going to throw this book on the sofa and go get a beer. Well, don't. This is easy, enormously useful, and eventually fun. Just subtract your age from 220, and you've got the conservative formula for your maximum heart rate. Easy-peasy. So, if you're forty, it's 220 minus forty or 180. If, like me, you are 72, it is 148. How hard was that, for Pete's sake?

Okay, now it's time for some third grade math: Figure out 60 percent of your max. (If you have trouble doing it in your head, just pull out your calculator and multiply your maximum heart rate by 0.6.) Write that number down. Better yet, memorize it. And remember this: *It is the sacred borderline between working out and fooling around.* A day when you get to 60 percent of your maximum heart rate and stay there for a significant period of time is a day you are working out; a day that you're not is a day on which you join the ranks of people volunteering to get old. Eventually, you will want to be able to go at 60 percent of your max for two or three hours, easy. But today, you may be

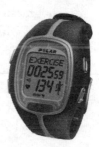

lucky to do it for fifteen minutes. Remember, whatever is serious for you is a serious workout. And another reminder: Don't forget to check with your doctor before you start any exercise regime.

ESTABLISHING A BASE

Before you start keeping this journal, you need to know how to find your waking heart rate and figure out your recovery rate.

* WAKING HEART RATE: Otherwise known as your resting heart rate, this is how fast your heart is beating before you get out of bed in the morning. So, first thing, just as you open your eyes, put on your heart rate monitor strap (which you have cleverly left on your bedside table), put the watch on your pillow, and almost go back to sleep. When you're so drowsy you can barely open your eyes, sneak a peek at the monitor. Or, if this is too complicated for you to handle, just put your index and middle fingers deep in your neck, next to your carotid artery, and count your heart beats while watching the second hand on your watch.

* RECOVERY RATE: This is the speed with which your heart rate drops in the sixty seconds after you've gone from peak exertion to a walk. So, if you've been working hard on your bike at, let's say, 80 percent of your max, just pedal easily while watching both your heart monitor and the second hand on your watch. Pedaling easily does not mean cruising along at a slower pace; it means drifting along with almost zero exertion. The instant your heart rate drops one beat (be sure to wait for it to go down one tick before you start timing, since it may go up before it starts to slow down), start timing. See how many beats per minute your heart rate drops in sixty seconds. (A glimpse at what you're going to learn later: Anything over 20 bpm

is satisfactory, but if you can get your recovery rate to 30 or 40, that's something to boast about.)

Okay, now we're ready to begin. And you're going to have to write down just a few more things. (Think of this as practice for journal-keeping. It's got to be a habit, after all.)

My weight: _____

My waking heart rate: _____

My recovery rate: _____

My normal aerobic activity (how many minutes spent on an elliptical machine, road bike, etc.): _____

How many days a week: _____

My normal weight activity (how much weight you lift, or what machines you use): _____

Frequency of normal weight activity (how many days a week): _____

If you're having a physical exam anytime soon, put all that dope down, too . . . your cholesterol numbers, blood pressure, and so on. That's an excellent idea, but don't wait for it to start keeping your log. Start today, do that later.

But remember this—medical numbers, especially choles- terol, may not change much with exercise. What does change dramatically is the implication of those numbers. So track them if it is of interest to you, but DO NOT get disappointed and stop exercising if the numbers don't change as you'd expect. You will be living longer with those exact same numbers if you are fit. *And the same thing goes for weight!!* Do not stop exercising if you do not lose the weight you expect. Neither Rome nor your gut was built (or destroyed) in a day.

KEEPING TRACK OF YOUR AEROBIC OR CARDIO WORKOUTS

A ll right, now we're down to the daily details, starting with aerobics. Remember, one size most assuredly does not fit all in this business. The goal, from the beginning, is to do an aerobic workout that is serious *for you*. The worst thing you can do is start hard and quit. Start slowly; honest. Then gradually crank it up. A hard walk or a very gentle bike ride (or a canter on the elliptical machine or treadmill) is fine for a long time if you're in seriously rotten shape. Like most people your age.

FINDING YOUR LEVEL

Level I: Over time, you will want to vary your aerobic workouts. Some days you'll want to tool along comfortably at the 60 percent level, which we call Level I or "long and slow." At that pace, you'll burn fat and build your aerobic base. It's about the best place to be for your general health and mobility.

Level II: When you're into it, you'll want to spend twenty to forty minutes at level II, which is 70–85 percent of your max. (Be sure to warm up for five minutes first, and to cool down for five minutes afterward. And sorry, neither the warm-up nor the cool-down counts as part of those twenty to forty minutes.) This kind of exertion is what we sometimes call the "endurance predator" level—a slightly wacky name meant to evoke our ancestral past, when we loped along the grassy plains looking for dinner. So don't worry: When you're moving at a clip, you're just living up to your design specs—while making your body faster and more powerful, and your state of mind more energetic and optimistic. Neat, huh?

Level III: For those of you who are already in good shape and want to push the envelope, you may want to think about interval training, sprinting, and so on. But this is not for the faint of heart—literally—and is beyond the scope of this journal. If you want to know more, you can see our website, www .youngernextyear.com.

PERCEIVED RATE OF EXERTION

If you refuse to get a heart rate monitor—and that would be dumb—you can tell very roughly where you are by figuring out your perceived rate of exertion. Level I is light exercise, equivalent for most people to a very brisk walk on level ground. If you are in very good shape, you probably can't get much above 50 percent of your max walking on the flat, but any kind of a hill will quickly get you over 60 percent. You can carry on a full conversation, and will work up a light sweat after the first twenty minutes or so. If you can't talk easily, and if you're really sweating, you've overshot the mark and should slow down. Remember that you lose the special benefits of "long and slow" if you go even a little bit too hard, so it is better to err on the light side.

Level II refers to a range of exercise that will take you from 70–85 percent of your maximum heart rate. In terms of perceived intensity, on the low end you'll begin to have trouble speaking in full sentences; at 85 percent, you'll be breathing deeply and comfortably, but you'll only be able to speak a couple of words at a time without running out of wind. It's important to realize that you have gone beyond your aerobic zone the moment you actually feel out of breath. Remember that the aerobic zone, by definition, is where you are still delivering oxygen to your tissues.

It makes sense to list, every day, what kind of aerobic exercise you did (biking, the elliptical machine, whatever), how many minutes you did it, and at what general level of intensity. But, remember, any week you do some kind of aerobics on four separate days is a good week. Consistency trumps passion. Consistency trumps everything.

In time you may want to get into the habit of having a really long and slow day—two or three hours on the bike, or a hike in the country at 60 percent of max. These long-and-slow days are not "required," but they sure are a good idea. Lots of serious endurance athletes do them—they're great at building your aerobic base. To say nothing of the fact that they are fun. It is *the* great thing to do at the end of a long and vexatious week! Trust me, after an hour and a half of biking or hiking or rowing, you won't remember what your office looks like.

FINDING YOUR TRUE MAXIMUM HEART RATE

By the way, the formula of 220-minus-your-age is roughly accurate, but each individual has his or her own maximum heart rate. As you go forward, your workouts will be more efficient if you take the time to find out yours. The simplest way to do this is to do a workout at the high end of Level II (as hard as you can sustain without feeling short of breath) for twenty minutes, then go up to your fastest pace for another two to three minutes (just barely shy of an all-out sprint). When you feel yourself start to run out of steam, go ahead and sprint for ten seconds and watch your heart monitor. Your heart rate will peak a few seconds *after* you finish sprinting. Write down the highest number. That's your maximum heart rate and you can use it instead of the formula. Because your max heart rate may increase somewhat as you get in better shape, and it may decrease somewhat with age, it's worth repeating this exercise every six months or so. Also, your maximum heart rate is a little different with different exercises (running, swimming, cycling, and canoeing will all produce mildly different maximum heart rates in the same individual). It's not worth worrying about unless you are serious about a couple of different endurance sports. If you are, then do the trial for each exercise.

Be sure to do the trials on days when you are well rested and well hydrated or you won't reach your true maximum. And be sure to clear this with your doctor ahead of time.

KEEPING TRACK OF WEIGHT WORK

L ifting weights is the single most important thing you can do to resist bone loss. And if that's not enough motivation: Who wants to have the muscles of their youth turn into the dusty drapery of old age? Or have joints that atrophy? So, go to the gym! For most people, two days of weight training per week is enough— your muscles need a day or even two to recover from a serious weight session. If you don't rest between sessions, it's all teardown and no buildup. Not good. And besides, you have to do aerobics four days a week no matter what.

While you should do a thorough strength workout, one that covers your lower body, your core (back and abs), and your upper body, you don't necessarily need to track every number. Most people benefit from keeping a list of the different exercises they do, and the weights they use, but for keeping track week by week, you can pick a couple of major exercises and just track them. Chris keeps track of 1) what he does on the leg press machine, 2) his pathetic effort at bicep curls with free weights, and 3) one of the core-strengthening machines that he likes.

But whatever you track, ALWAYS REMEMBER with strength training that you are doing it for your joints, not your muscles. Instead of asking, "Are my legs strong enough to go from pressing 200 pounds to 220 pounds?" (to which the answer is "yes"), ask yourself, "Are my knees strong enough to go up to 220 pounds?" and realize that the answer is probably "maybe." Your muscles get strong about three times faster than your joints, so you can easily get strong enough to pull your joints apart if you progress at the pace of your muscles.

That's why we strongly recommend that you use a trainer to get started with weights. It's easy to hurt yourself. But if you concentrate on good form, and listen to your joints instead of your muscles, you should be fine. And in the long run, everything will feel better because of strength training.

KEEPING TRACK OF FOOD

In case you haven't memorized "Harry's Rules" yet, let us remind you about Rule #5. It's "Quit Eating Crap." Take a moment to absorb that thought, and then realize that tracking what you eat (and how much of it you're eating) is probably the best way to avoid the bad stuff. It's also a great way to keep from overeating. Again, don't go overboard—just keep a rough log of the kinds of portions you're eating and how much of the dreaded *crap* you eat. Also booze and wine, if you drink, because you've got to keep track of portions there.

Make a list right now of the crap you love . . . your own Top Ten of food to avoid. Here's Chris's: Bread and butter; french fries; pasta; pizza; Chinese take-out of almost all kinds; white rice; fast-food burgers; crackers and popcorn and chips and tacos and all the rest of the nibbles family. The simple version? Don't eat white stuff!

Harry is alarmingly virtuous. When asked for his "crap" list, listen to what he said: "I don't have as much trouble with this as Chris does, because, frankly, I don't care that much about food. I am equally happy with a salad or a doughnut, so for me it's a function of being sure healthy food shows up on my plate as often as possible. I have found it a great relief to simply make breakfast and lunch meals I don't think about. Translation? Breakfast is a cup of coffee, two bananas, and a bowl of high-fiber cereal with skim milk. I neither love it, nor hate it; I simply eat it."

Harry goes on: "Lunch is cashew or almond nut butter (I got sick of peanut butter) and jelly on true whole grain bread, plus two apples. Again, I don't care either way—it is just convenient and healthy. Dinner always involves a salad, and most of the time is fairly healthy stuff, but if I have some crap now and then, at least it is because I actually wanted it, not because it was the default setting. Chris finds this approach horrifying; I find it relaxing and very effective. But it does depend on having a relatively neutral attitude toward food!"

NOW IT'S YOUR TURN

We're assuming the rest of you aren't so virtuous as Harry about the foods you eat, so now it's your turn to write down the foods that call your name. Be honest!

THE FOODS I NEED TO AVOID

_____

_____

_____

_____

_____

_____

_____

_____

_____

KEEPING TRACK OF CONNECTION AND COMMITMENT EFFORTS

Connecting with other people and doing things you're passionate about are probably as important as anything. We are mammals, and we are hardwired to work and play in packs and groups. If we don't, we get sick. Literally. As we get older, a lot of us tend to get more isolated. Bad, bad idea. Gotta make a serious effort to stay involved with—and care about—other people and groups. Sounds goody-goody, but it's not.

Connecting to others and giving back to your community are such nebulous goals that they risk falling into the New Year's resolution category. And they don't exactly lend themselves to journalizing, but give it a shot. Set a goal for how many times a week you want to reach out to your friends via phone or e-mail. Come up with social events—movie nights, workout sessions, whatever—that you might organize. And then keep track of how you do. It will serve as a daily, or at least a weekly, reminder that these things really matter.

The same goes for community and spiritual commitments. They don't need to take up much space in the journal, but put yourself on the hook for writing down what you are doing for the broader good. It will pull you forward—and upward—as much as exercise can.

Okay, that's the deal. Very simple, very easy, and very, very important. As sailors have known for a thousand years, keep a good log and you stand a radically better chance of getting where you want to go. And of not falling off the edge of the world. If you find yourself missing days, write less, but write something every day. No matter what. Forever.

The Workout Journal

Turn Back Your Biological Clock

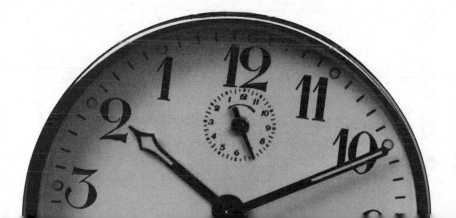

1
week

Exercise & Diet Plan for the Week

	MONDAY	TUESDAY	WEDNESDAY	THURSDAY	FRIDAY	SATURDAY	SUNDAY
CARDIO							
WEIGHTS							

Weight at beginning of week: _____ Weight at end of week: _____

Goals for the week: _____

Ideas for caring, connecting, committing: _____

CHRIS SAYS: DON'T VOLUNTEER!

Here's our core message: 70% of aging is voluntary . . . as is 50% of all the serious illnesses and accidents that knock you down after forty-five or fifty. *So don't volunteer.* Instead, send your body a message to stop decaying. How? By doing three things: 1) exercise, 2) connect with others, and 3) quit eating crap. But the first and most important, always, is exercise *six days a week.* That's hard. So start today. And never stop. Ever. If you're in decent shape, go for it. If not, read on . . .

Monday ___ | | |

How was your night?

Morning mood: _____ Resting Heart Rate: _____

E X E R C I S E

CARDIO

Time and/or distance: _____ Level: _____ Heart Rate Max: _____ Recovery: _____

STRENGTH: UPPER BODY & BACK		STRENGTH: LEGS & ABS	
1:	Reps:	1:	Reps:
2:	Reps:	2:	Reps:
3:	Reps:	3:	Reps:
4:	Reps:	4:	Reps:
5:	Reps:	5:	Reps:

F O O D

Breakfast:

Lunch:

Dinner:

Snacks: _____ Crap: _____ Booze: _____

L I F E

Caring, connecting, committing:

How did you do? ☐ Amazing ☐ Not Bad ☐ Shameful

Plans for tomorrow:

Tuesday ___ | | |

How was your night?

Morning mood: Resting Heart Rate:

EXERCISE

CARDIO

Time and/or distance: Level: Heart Rate Max: Recovery:

STRENGTH: UPPER BODY & BACK		STRENGTH: LEGS & ABS	
1:	Reps:	1:	Reps:
2:	Reps:	2:	Reps:
3:	Reps:	3:	Reps:
4:	Reps:	4:	Reps:
5:	Reps:	5:	Reps:

FOOD

Breakfast:

Lunch:

Dinner:

Snacks: Crap: Booze:

LIFE

Caring, connecting, committing:

How did you do? ☐ Amazing ☐ Not Bad ☐ Shameful

Plans for tomorrow:

Wednesday ___ | | |

How was your night?

Morning mood: Resting Heart Rate:

EXERCISE

CARDIO

Time and/or distance: Level: Heart Rate Max: Recovery:

STRENGTH: UPPER BODY & BACK		STRENGTH: LEGS & ABS	
1:	Reps:	1:	Reps:
2:	Reps:	2:	Reps:
3:	Reps.	3:	Reps:
4:	Reps:	4:	Reps:
5:	Reps:	5:	Reps:

FOOD

Breakfast:

Lunch:

Dinner:

Snacks: Crap: Booze:

LIFE

Caring, connecting, committing:

How did you do? ☐ Amazing ☐ Not Bad ☐ Shameful

Plans for tomorrow:

Thursday___|___|___|

How was your night?

Morning mood: Resting Heart Rate:

E X E R C I S E

CARDIO

Time and/or distance: Level: Heart Rate Max: Recovery:

STRENGTH: UPPER BODY & BACK		**STRENGTH: LEGS & ABS**	
1:	Reps:	1:	Reps:
2:	Reps:	2:	Reps:
3:	Reps:	3:	Reps:
4:	Reps:	4:	Reps:
5:	Reps:	5:	Reps:

F O O D

Breakfast:

Lunch:

Dinner:

Snacks: Crap: Booze:

L I F E

Caring, connecting, committing:

How did you do?   ☐ Amazing   ☐ Not Bad   ☐ Shameful

Plans for tomorrow:

Friday___|___|___|

How was your night?

Morning mood: Resting Heart Rate:

E X E R C I S E

CARDIO

Time and/or distance: Level: Heart Rate Max: Recovery:

STRENGTH: UPPER BODY & BACK		**STRENGTH: LEGS & ABS**	
1:	Reps:	1:	Reps:
2:	Reps:	2:	Reps:
3:	Reps:	3:	Reps:
4:	Reps:	4:	Reps:
5:	Reps:	5:	Reps:

F O O D

Breakfast:

Lunch:

Dinner:

Snacks: Crap: Booze:

L I F E

Caring, connecting, committing:

How did you do?   ☐ Amazing   ☐ Not Bad   ☐ Shameful

Plans for tomorrow:

Saturday ___ | | |

How was your night?

Morning mood: Resting Heart Rate:

E X E R C I S E

CARDIO

Time and/or distance: Level: Heart Rate Max: Recovery:

STRENGTH: UPPER BODY & BACK		**STRENGTH: LEGS & ABS**	
1:	Reps:	1:	Reps:
2:	Reps:	2:	Reps:
3:	Reps:	3:	Reps:
4:	Reps:	4:	Reps:
5:	Reps:	5:	Reps:

F O O D

Breakfast:

Lunch:

Dinner:

Snacks: Crap: Booze:

L I F E

Caring, connecting, committing:

How did you do?   ☐ Amazing   ☐ Not Bad   ☐ Shameful

Plans for tomorrow:

Sunday ___ | | |

How was your night?

Morning mood: Resting Heart Rate:

E X E R C I S E

CARDIO

Time and/or distance: Level: Heart Rate Max: Recovery:

STRENGTH: UPPER BODY & BACK		**STRENGTH: LEGS & ABS**	
1:	Reps:	1:	Reps:
2:	Reps:	2:	Reps:
3:	Reps:	3:	Reps:
4:	Reps:	4:	Reps:
5:	Reps:	5:	Reps:

F O O D

Breakfast:

Lunch:

Dinner:

Snacks: Crap: Booze:

L I F E

Caring, connecting, committing:

How did you do?   ☐ Amazing   ☐ Not Bad   ☐ Shameful

Plans for tomorrow:

2 week Exercise & Diet Plan for the Week

	MONDAY	TUESDAY	WEDNESDAY	THURSDAY	FRIDAY	SATURDAY	SUNDAY
CARDIO							
WEIGHTS							

Weight at beginning of week: _____ Weight at end of week: _____

Goals for the week:

Ideas for caring, connecting, committing:

HARRY SAYS: **FIND YOUR INNER ATHLETE**

Even if you haven't exercised in years (or ever), take heart. Buried inside *all of us* lies an athlete. Still, if you are deeply "de-conditioned," it may take months to find the brute within. Translation? If you're in awful shape, jump into daily exercise with both feet, but make it gentle. For the first month, do ten minutes a day of light walking, or the equivalent of an elliptical trainer or stationary bike. Up your daily exercise a little bit each week until you reach thirty minutes a day. It doesn't matter if that takes a month or a year. As long as you show up, you are triumphant!

Monday | | |

How was your night? _____

Morning mood: _____ Resting Heart Rate: _____

EXERCISE

CARDIO

Time and/or distance: _____ Level: _____ Heart Rate Max: _____ Recovery: _____

STRENGTH: UPPER BODY & BACK		STRENGTH: LEGS & ABS	
1:	Reps:	1:	Reps:
2:	Reps:	2:	Reps:
3:	Reps:	3:	Reps:
4:	Reps:	4:	Reps:
5:	Reps:	5:	Reps:

FOOD

Breakfast:

Lunch:

Dinner:

Snacks: _____ Crap: _____ Booze: _____

LIFE

Caring, connecting, committing:

How did you do? ☐ Amazing ☐ Not Bad ☐ Shameful

Plans for tomorrow:

Tuesday___ | | |

How was your night?

Morning mood: Resting Heart Rate:

E X E R C I S E

CARDIO

Time and/or distance: Level: Heart Rate Max: Recovery:

STRENGTH: UPPER BODY & BACK		STRENGTH: LEGS & ABS	
1:	Reps:	1:	Reps:
2:	Reps:	2:	Reps:
3:	Reps:	3:	Reps:
4:	Reps:	4:	Reps:
5:	Reps:	5:	Reps:

F O O D

Breakfast:

Lunch:

Dinner:

Snacks: Crap: Booze:

L I F E

Caring, connecting, committing:

How did you do? ☐ Amazing ☐ Not Bad ☐ Shameful

Plans for tomorrow:

Wednesday___ | | |

How was your night?

Morning mood: Resting Heart Rate:

E X E R C I S E

CARDIO

Time and/or distance: Level: Heart Rate Max: Recovery:

STRENGTH: UPPER BODY & BACK		STRENGTH: LEGS & ABS	
1:	Reps:	1:	Reps:
2:	Reps:	2:	Reps:
3:	Reps:	3:	Reps:
4:	Reps:	4:	Reps:
5:	Reps:	5:	Reps:

F O O D

Breakfast:

Lunch:

Dinner:

Snacks: Crap: Booze:

L I F E

Caring, connecting, committing:

How did you do? ☐ Amazing ☐ Not Bad ☐ Shameful

Plans for tomorrow:

Thursday___|__|__|

How was your night?

Morning mood: Resting Heart Rate:

EXERCISE

CARDIO

Time and/or distance: Level: Heart Rate Max: Recovery:

STRENGTH: UPPER BODY & BACK		STRENGTH: LEGS & ABS	
1:	Reps:	1:	Reps:
2:	Reps:	2:	Reps:
3:	Reps:	3:	Reps:
4:	Reps:	4:	Reps:
5:	Reps:	5:	Reps:

FOOD

Breakfast:

Lunch:

Dinner:

Snacks: Crap: Booze:

LIFE

Caring, connecting, committing:

How did you do? ☐ Amazing ☐ Not Bad ☐ Shameful

Plans for tomorrow:

Friday___|__|__|

How was your night?

Morning mood: Resting Heart Rate:

EXERCISE

CARDIO

Time and/or distance: Level: Heart Rate Max: Recovery:

STRENGTH: UPPER BODY & BACK		STRENGTH: LEGS & ABS	
1:	Reps:	1:	Reps:
2:	Reps:	2:	Reps:
3:	Reps:	3:	Reps:
4:	Reps:	4:	Reps:
5:	Reps:	5:	Reps:

FOOD

Breakfast:

Lunch:

Dinner:

Snacks: Crap: Booze:

LIFE

Caring, connecting, committing:

How did you do? ☐ Amazing ☐ Not Bad ☐ Shameful

Plans for tomorrow:

Saturday___ | | |

How was your night?

Morning mood: Resting Heart Rate:

EXERCISE

CARDIO

Time and/or distance: Level: Heart Rate Max: Recovery:

STRENGTH: UPPER BODY & BACK		STRENGTH: LEGS & ABS	
1:	Reps:	1:	Reps:
2:	Reps:	2:	Reps:
3:	Reps:	3:	Reps:
4:	Reps:	4:	Reps:
5:	Reps:	5:	Reps:

FOOD

Breakfast:

Lunch:

Dinner:

Snacks: Crap: Booze:

LIFE

Caring, connecting, committing:

How did you do? ☐ Amazing ☐ Not Bad ☐ Shameful

Plans for tomorrow:

Sunday___ | | |

How was your night?

Morning mood: Resting Heart Rate:

EXERCISE

CARDIO

Time and/or distance: Level: Heart Rate Max: Recovery:

STRENGTH: UPPER BODY & BACK		STRENGTH: LEGS & ABS	
1:	Reps:	1:	Reps:
2:	Reps:	2:	Reps:
3:	Reps:	3:	Reps:
4:	Reps:	4:	Reps:
5:	Reps:	5:	Reps:

FOOD

Breakfast:

Lunch:

Dinner:

Snacks: Crap: Booze:

LIFE

Caring, connecting, committing:

How did you do? ☐ Amazing ☐ Not Bad ☐ Shameful

Plans for tomorrow:

3 week Exercise & Diet Plan for the Week

	MONDAY	TUESDAY	WEDNESDAY	THURSDAY	FRIDAY	SATURDAY	SUNDAY
CARDIO							
WEIGHTS							

Weight at beginning of week: _____ Weight at end of week: _____

Goals for the week:

Ideas for caring, connecting, committing:

CHRIS SAYS: LEARN TO KEDGE

When sailors got becalmed and were drifting toward the rocks, they would literally pull themselves forward (using a small boat to set a small anchor) to get out of danger. They called it kedging. And that's what you have to do when you are tempted to say the hell with it and never exercise again. Try a weeklong bike trip. Go skiing. Book yourself into a serious spa. Getting ready for such a trip is a serious motivator—the trip itself gets you in better shape, and the memory of it keeps you going for months after.

Monday _____

How was your night?

Morning mood: _____ Resting Heart Rate: _____

E X E R C I S E

CARDIO

Time and/or distance: _____ Level: _____ Heart Rate Max: _____ Recovery: _____

STRENGTH: UPPER BODY & BACK		STRENGTH: LEGS & ABS	
1:	Reps:	1:	Reps:
2:	Reps:	2:	Reps:
3:	Reps:	3:	Reps:
4:	Reps:	4:	Reps:
5:	Reps:	5:	Reps:

F O O D

Breakfast:

Lunch:

Dinner:

Snacks: _____ Crap: _____ Booze: _____

L I F E

Caring, connecting, committing:

How did you do? ☐ Amazing ☐ Not Bad ☐ Shameful

Plans for tomorrow:

Tuesday ___ | | |

How was your night?

Morning mood: Resting Heart Rate:

EXERCISE

CARDIO

Time and/or distance: Level: Heart Rate Max: Recovery:

STRENGTH: UPPER BODY & BACK		STRENGTH: LEGS & ABS	
1:	Reps:	1:	Reps:
2:	Reps:	2:	Reps:
3:	Reps:	3:	Reps:
4:	Reps:	4:	Reps:
5:	Reps:	5:	Reps:

FOOD

Breakfast:

Lunch:

Dinner:

Snacks: Crap: Booze:

LIFE

Caring, connecting, committing:

How did you do?   ☐ Amazing ☐ Not Bad ☐ Shameful

Plans for tomorrow:

Wednesday ___ | | |

How was your night?

Morning mood: Resting Heart Rate:

EXERCISE

CARDIO

Time and/or distance: Level: Heart Rate Max: Recovery:

STRENGTH: UPPER BODY & BACK		STRENGTH: LEGS & ABS	
1:	Reps:	1:	Reps:
2:	Reps:	2:	Reps:
3:	Reps:	3:	Reps:
4:	Reps:	4:	Reps:
5:	Reps:	5:	Reps:

FOOD

Breakfast:

Lunch:

Dinner:

Snacks: Crap: Booze:

LIFE

Caring, connecting, committing:

How did you do?   ☐ Amazing ☐ Not Bad ☐ Shameful

Plans for tomorrow:

Thursday ⎿ ⎿ ⎿

How was your night?

Morning mood: Resting Heart Rate:

E X E R C I S E

CARDIO

Time and/or distance: Level: Heart Rate Max: Recovery:

STRENGTH: UPPER BODY & BACK		STRENGTH: LEGS & ABS	
1:	Reps:	1:	Reps:
2:	Reps:	2:	Reps:
3:	Reps:	3:	Reps:
4:	Reps:	4:	Reps:
5:	Reps:	5:	Reps:

F O O D

Breakfast:

Lunch:

Dinner:

Snacks: Crap: Booze:

L I F E

Caring, connecting, committing:

How did you do?   ☐ Amazing   ☐ Not Bad   ☐ Shameful

Plans for tomorrow:

Friday ⎿ ⎿ ⎿

How was your night?

Morning mood: Resting Heart Rate:

E X E R C I S E

CARDIO

Time and/or distance: Level: Heart Rate Max: Recovery:

STRENGTH: UPPER BODY & BACK		STRENGTH: LEGS & ABS	
1:	Reps:	1:	Reps:
2:	Reps:	2:	Reps:
3:	Reps:	3:	Reps:
4:	Reps:	4:	Reps:
5:	Reps:	5:	Reps:

F O O D

Breakfast:

Lunch:

Dinner:

Snacks: Crap: Booze:

L I F E

Caring, connecting, committing:

How did you do?   ☐ Amazing   ☐ Not Bad   ☐ Shameful

Plans for tomorrow:

Saturday___|__|__|

	How was your night?	
	Morning mood:	Resting Heart Rate:

E X E R C I S E

CARDIO

Time and/or distance: Level: Heart Rate Max: Recovery:

STRENGTH: UPPER BODY & BACK		STRENGTH: LEGS & ABS	
1:	Reps:	1:	Reps:
2:	Reps:	2:	Reps:
3:	Reps:	3:	Reps:
4:	Reps:	4:	Reps:
5:	Reps:	5:	Reps:

F O O D

Breakfast:

Lunch:

Dinner:

Snacks: Crap: Booze:

L I F E

Caring, connecting, committing:

How did you do?   ☐ Amazing ☐ Not Bad ☐ Shameful

Plans for tomorrow:

Sunday___|__|__|

	How was your night?	
	Morning mood:	Resting Heart Rate:

E X E R C I S E

CARDIO

Time and/or distance: Level: Heart Rate Max: Recovery:

STRENGTH: UPPER BODY & BACK		STRENGTH: LEGS & ABS	
1:	Reps:	1:	Reps:
2:	Reps:	2:	Reps:
3:	Reps:	3:	Reps:
4:	Reps:	4:	Reps:
5:	Reps:	5:	Reps:

F O O D

Breakfast:

Lunch:

Dinner:

Snacks: Crap: Booze:

L I F E

Caring, connecting, committing:

How did you do?   ☐ Amazing ☐ Not Bad ☐ Shameful

Plans for tomorrow:

Exercise & Diet Plan for the Week

	MONDAY	TUESDAY	WEDNESDAY	THURSDAY	FRIDAY	SATURDAY	SUNDAY
CARDIO							
WEIGHTS							

Weight at beginning of week: Weight at end of week:

Goals for the week:

Ideas for caring, connecting, committing:

CHRIS SAYS: JOIN A GYM

You may hate gyms. Fine. Join one anyway. You'd rather work out on your bike? Great. Join a gym. You need one for those days when it's too awful to go outside. You need one for the weight machines and the trainers. You need one for the classes. You need one for the community. So join a gym. It's indispensable. Honest.

Monday _ | | |

How was your night?

Morning mood: Resting Heart Rate:

E X E R C I S E

CARDIO

Time and/or distance: Level: Heart Rate Max: Recovery:

STRENGTH: UPPER BODY & BACK		**STRENGTH: LEGS & ABS**	
1:	Reps:	1:	Reps:
2:	Reps:	2:	Reps:
3:	Reps:	3:	Reps:
4:	Reps:	4:	Reps:
5:	Reps:	5:	Reps:

F O O D

Breakfast:

Lunch:

Dinner:

Snacks: Crap: Booze:

L I F E

Caring, connecting, committing:

How did you do? ☐ Amazing ☐ Not Bad ☐ Shameful

Plans for tomorrow:

Tuesday___|__|__|

How was your night?

Morning mood: Resting Heart Rate:

E X E R C I S E

CARDIO

Time and/or distance: Level: Heart Rate Max: Recovery:

STRENGTH: UPPER BODY & BACK		**STRENGTH: LEGS & ABS**	
1:	Reps:	1:	Reps:
2:	Reps:	2:	Reps:
3:	Reps:	3:	Reps:
4:	Reps:	4:	Reps:
5:	Reps:	5:	Reps:

F O O D

Breakfast:

Lunch:

Dinner:

Snacks: Crap: Booze:

L I F E

Caring, connecting, committing:

How did you do?   ☐ Amazing   ☐ Not Bad   ☐ Shameful

Plans for tomorrow:

Wednesday___|__|__|

How was your night?

Morning mood: Resting Heart Rate:

E X E R C I S E

CARDIO

Time and/or distance: Level: Heart Rate Max: Recovery:

STRENGTH: UPPER BODY & BACK		**STRENGTH: LEGS & ABS**	
1:	Reps:	1:	Reps:
2:	Reps:	2:	Reps:
3:	Reps:	3:	Reps:
4:	Reps:	4:	Reps:
5:	Reps:	5:	Reps:

F O O D

Breakfast:

Lunch:

Dinner:

Snacks: Crap: Booze:

L I F E

Caring, connecting, committing:

How did you do?   ☐ Amazing   ☐ Not Bad   ☐ Shameful

Plans for tomorrow:

Thursday ___|___|___

How was your night?

Morning mood: Resting Heart Rate:

EXERCISE

CARDIO

Time and/or distance: Level: Heart Rate Max: Recovery:

STRENGTH: UPPER BODY & BACK		STRENGTH: LEGS & ABS	
1:	Reps:	1:	Reps:
2:	Reps:	2:	Reps:
3:	Reps:	3:	Reps:
4:	Reps:	4:	Reps:
5:	Reps:	5:	Reps:

FOOD

Breakfast:

Lunch:

Dinner:

Snacks: Crap: Booze:

LIFE

Caring, connecting, committing:

How did you do?   ☐ Amazing   ☐ Not Bad   ☐ Shameful

Plans for tomorrow:

Friday ___|___|___

How was your night?

Morning mood: Resting Heart Rate:

EXERCISE

CARDIO

Time and/or distance: Level: Heart Rate Max: Recovery:

STRENGTH: UPPER BODY & BACK		STRENGTH: LEGS & ABS	
1:	Reps:	1:	Reps:
2:	Reps:	2:	Reps:
3:	Reps:	3:	Reps:
4:	Reps:	4:	Reps:
5:	Reps:	5:	Reps:

FOOD

Breakfast:

Lunch:

Dinner:

Snacks: Crap: Booze:

LIFE

Caring, connecting, committing:

How did you do?   ☐ Amazing   ☐ Not Bad   ☐ Shameful

Plans for tomorrow:

Saturday _____ | | |

	How was your night?	
	Morning mood:	Resting Heart Rate:

E X E R C I S E

CARDIO

Time and/or distance:	Level:	Heart Rate Max:	Recovery:

STRENGTH: UPPER BODY & BACK		STRENGTH: LEGS & ABS	
1:	Reps:	1:	Reps:
2:	Reps:	2:	Reps:
3:	Reps:	3:	Reps:
4:	Reps:	4:	Reps:
5:	Reps:	5:	Reps:

F O O D

Breakfast:

Lunch:

Dinner:

Snacks:	Crap:	Booze.

L I F E

Caring, connecting, committing:

How did you do? ☐ Amazing ☐ Not Bad ☐ Shameful

Plans for tomorrow:

Sunday _____ | | |

	How was your night?	
	Morning mood:	Resting Heart Rate:

E X E R C I S E

CARDIO

Time and/or distance:	Level:	Heart Rate Max:	Recovery:

STRENGTH: UPPER BODY & BACK		STRENGTH: LEGS & ABS	
1:	Reps:	1:	Reps:
2:	Reps:	2:	Reps:
3:	Reps:	3:	Reps:
4:	Reps:	4:	Reps:
5:	Reps:	5:	Reps:

F O O D

Breakfast:

Lunch:

Dinner:

Snacks:	Crap:	Booze:

L I F E

Caring, connecting, committing:

How did you do? ☐ Amazing ☐ Not Bad ☐ Shameful

Plans for tomorrow:

5 week

Exercise & Diet Plan for the Week

	MONDAY	TUESDAY	WEDNESDAY	THURSDAY	FRIDAY	SATURDAY	SUNDAY
CARDIO							
WEIGHTS							

Weight at beginning of week: _____   Weight at end of week: _____

Goals for the week: _____

Ideas for caring, connecting, committing: _____

HARRY SAYS: ENJOY YOUR WEEKENDS

Very few of us have time for this during the week, but devoting one day a week to a very long and slow workout (two to three hours at 60% of your max, which, for most people, translates into being outdoors walking or biking), is a serious treat. Enjoy yourself. You deserve it.

Monthy ___|___|___

How was your night? _____
Morning mood: _____   Resting Heart Rate: _____

E X E R C I S E

CARDIO

Time and/or distance: _____ Level: _____   Heart Rate Max: _____   Recovery: _____

STRENGTH: UPPER BODY & BACK		**STRENGTH: LEGS & ABS**	
1:	Reps:	1:	Reps:
2:	Reps:	2:	Reps:
3:	Reps:	3:	Reps:
4:	Reps:	4:	Reps:
5:	Reps:	5:	Reps:

F O O D

Breakfast:

Lunch:

Dinner:

Snacks: _____   Crap: _____   Booze: _____

L I F E

Caring, connecting, committing:

How did you do?   ☐ Amazing   ☐ Not Bad   ☐ Shameful

Plans for tomorrow:

Tuesday ___ | | |

How was your night?

Morning mood: Resting Heart Rate:

EXERCISE

CARDIO

Time and/or distance: Level: Heart Rate Max: Recovery:

STRENGTH: UPPER BODY & BACK		STRENGTH: LEGS & ABS	
1:	Reps:	1:	Reps:
2:	Reps:	2:	Reps:
3:	Reps:	3:	Reps:
4:	Reps:	4:	Reps:
5:	Reps:	5:	Reps:

FOOD

Breakfast:

Lunch:

Dinner:

Snacks: Crap: Booze:

LIFE

Caring, connecting, committing:

How did you do? ☐ Amazing ☐ Not Bad ☐ Shameful

Plans for tomorrow:

Wednesday ___ | | |

How was your night?

Morning mood: Resting Heart Rate:

EXERCISE

CARDIO

Time and/or distance: Level: Heart Rate Max: Recovery:

STRENGTH: UPPER BODY & BACK		STRENGTH: LEGS & ABS	
1:	Reps:	1:	Reps:
2:	Reps:	2:	Reps:
3:	Reps:	3:	Reps:
4:	Reps:	4:	Reps:
5:	Reps:	5:	Reps:

FOOD

Breakfast:

Lunch:

Dinner:

Snacks: Crap: Booze:

LIFE

Caring, connecting, committing:

How did you do? ☐ Amazing ☐ Not Bad ☐ Shameful

Plans for tomorrow:

Thursday | | |

How was your night?

Morning mood: Resting Heart Rate:

E X E R C I S E

CARDIO

Time and/or distance: Level: Heart Rate Max: Recovery:

STRENGTH: UPPER BODY & BACK		STRENGTH: LEGS & ABS	
1:	Reps:	1:	Reps:
2:	Reps:	2:	Reps:
3:	Reps:	3:	Reps:
4:	Reps:	4:	Reps:
5:	Reps:	5:	Reps:

F O O D

Breakfast:

Lunch:

Dinner:

Snacks: Crap: Booze:

L I F E

Caring, connecting, committing:

How did you do?   ☐ Amazing ☐ Not Bad ☐ Shameful

Plans for tomorrow:

Friday | | |

How was your night?

Morning mood: Resting Heart Rate:

E X E R C I S E

CARDIO

Time and/or distance: Level: Heart Rate Max: Recovery:

STRENGTH: UPPER BODY & BACK		STRENGTH: LEGS & ABS	
1:	Reps:	1:	Reps:
2:	Reps:	2:	Reps:
3:	Reps:	3:	Reps:
4:	Reps:	4:	Reps:
5:	Reps:	5:	Reps:

F O O D

Breakfast:

Lunch:

Dinner:

Snacks: Crap: Booze:

L I F E

Caring, connecting, committing:

How did you do?   ☐ Amazing ☐ Not Bad ☐ Shameful

Plans for tomorrow:

Saturday___|___|___|

How was your night?

Morning mood: Resting Heart Rate:

EXERCISE

CARDIO

Time and/or distance: Level: Heart Rate Max: Recovery:

STRENGTH: UPPER BODY & BACK		STRENGTH: LEGS & ABS	
1:	Reps:	1:	Reps:
2:	Reps:	2:	Reps:
3:	Reps:	3:	Reps:
4:	Reps:	4:	Reps:
5:	Reps:	5:	Reps:

FOOD

Breakfast:

Lunch:

Dinner:

Snacks: Crap: Booze:

LIFE

Caring, connecting, committing:

How did you do?   ☐ Amazing   ☐ Not Bad   ☐ Shameful

Plans for tomorrow:

Sunday___|___|___|

How was your night?

Morning mood: Resting Heart Rate:

EXERCISE

CARDIO

Time and/or distance: Level: Heart Rate Max: Recovery:

STRENGTH: UPPER BODY & BACK		STRENGTH: LEGS & ABS	
1:	Reps:	1:	Reps:
2:	Reps:	2:	Reps:
3:	Reps:	3:	Reps:
4:	Reps:	4:	Reps:
5:	Reps:	5:	Reps:

FOOD

Breakfast:

Lunch:

Dinner:

Snacks: Crap: Booze:

LIFE

Caring, connecting, committing:

How did you do?   ☐ Amazing   ☐ Not Bad   ☐ Shameful

Plans for tomorrow:

6 week

Exercise & Diet Plan for the Week

	MONDAY	TUESDAY	WEDNESDAY	THURSDAY	FRIDAY	SATURDAY	SUNDAY
CARDIO							
WEIGHTS							

Weight at beginning of week: _____ Weight at end of week: _____

Goals for the week:

Ideas for caring, connecting, committing:

CHRIS SAYS: GET UP!

Create a pattern early on. Even if you aren't a morning person, try getting out
of bed, first thing, and going to the gym (or out on your bike, or whatever) . . .
before other responsibilities lay claim to your day. Don't think about it. Just go
for it. Who wants to get tangled up in endless (and often self-defeating) decision-
making every day? Got it? Good. Get up. Or, if you're built that way, make
lunchtime exercise your pattern. Or do it just before supper. But set a pattern.

Monday __ |__|__|

How was your night?

Morning mood: _____ Resting Heart Rate:

E X E R C I S E

CARDIO

Time and/or distance: _____ Level: _____ Heart Rate Max: _____ Recovery:

STRENGTH: UPPER BODY & BACK		**STRENGTH: LEGS & ABS**	
1:	Reps:	1:	Reps:
2:	Reps:	2:	Reps:
3:	Reps:	3:	Reps:
4:	Reps:	4:	Reps:
5:	Reps:	5:	Reps:

F O O D

Breakfast:

Lunch:

Dinner:

Snacks: _____ Crap: _____ Booze:

L I F E

Caring, connecting, committing:

How did you do? ☐ Amazing ☐ Not Bad ☐ Shameful

Plans for tomorrow:

Tuesday _|_|_|

How was your night?

Morning mood: Resting Heart Rate:

EXERCISE

CARDIO

Time and/or distance: Level: Heart Rate Max: Recovery:

STRENGTH: UPPER BODY & BACK		STRENGTH: LEGS & ABS	
1:	Reps:	1:	Reps:
2:	Reps:	2:	Reps:
3:	Reps:	3:	Reps:
4:	Reps:	4:	Reps:
5:	Reps:	5:	Reps:

FOOD

Breakfast:

Lunch:

Dinner:

Snacks: Crap: Booze:

LIFE

Caring, connecting, committing:

How did you do? ☐ Amazing ☐ Not Bad ☐ Shameful

Plans for tomorrow:

Wednesday _|_|_|

How was your night?

Morning mood: Resting Heart Rate:

EXERCISE

CARDIO

Time and/or distance: Level: Heart Rate Max: Recovery:

STRENGTH: UPPER BODY & BACK		STRENGTH: LEGS & ABS	
1:	Reps:	1:	Reps:
2:	Reps:	2:	Reps:
3:	Reps:	3:	Reps:
4:	Reps:	4:	Reps:
5:	Reps:	5:	Reps:

FOOD

Breakfast:

Lunch:

Dinner:

Snacks: Crap: Booze:

LIFE

Caring, connecting, committing:

How did you do? ☐ Amazing ☐ Not Bad ☐ Shameful

Plans for tomorrow:

Thursday ___ | | |

How was your night?

Morning mood: Resting Heart Rate:

E X E R C I S E

CARDIO

Time and/or distance: Level: Heart Rate Max: Recovery:

STRENGTH: UPPER BODY & BACK		**STRENGTH: LEGS & ABS**	
1:	Reps:	1:	Reps:
2:	Reps:	2:	Reps:
3:	Reps:	3:	Reps:
4:	Reps:	4:	Reps:
5:	Reps:	5:	Reps:

F O O D

Breakfast:

Lunch:

Dinner:

Snacks: Crap: Booze:

L I F E

Caring, connecting, committing:

How did you do?   ☐ Amazing ☐ Not Bad ☐ Shameful

Plans for tomorrow:

Friday ___ | | |

How was your night?

Morning mood: Resting Heart Rate:

E X E R C I S E

CARDIO

Time and/or distance: Level: Heart Rate Max: Recovery:

STRENGTH: UPPER BODY & BACK		**STRENGTH: LEGS & ABS**	
1:	Reps:	1:	Reps:
2:	Reps:	2:	Reps:
3:	Reps:	3:	Reps:
4:	Reps:	4:	Reps:
5:	Reps:	5:	Reps:

F O O D

Breakfast:

Lunch:

Dinner:

Snacks: Crap: Booze:

L I F E

Caring, connecting, committing:

How did you do?   ☐ Amazing ☐ Not Bad ☐ Shameful

Plans for tomorrow:

Saturday _|_|_

How was your night?

Morning mood: Resting Heart Rate:

EXERCISE

CARDIO

Time and/or distance: Level: Heart Rate Max: Recovery:

STRENGTH: UPPER BODY & BACK		STRENGTH: LEGS & ABS	
1:	Reps:	1:	Reps:
2:	Reps:	2:	Reps:
3:	Reps:	3:	Reps:
4:	Reps:	4:	Reps:
5:	Reps:	5:	Reps:

FOOD

Breakfast:

Lunch:

Dinner:

Snacks: Crap: Booze:

LIFE

Caring, connecting, committing:

How did you do? ☐ Amazing ☐ Not Bad ☐ Shameful

Plans for tomorrow:

Sunday _|_|_

How was your night?

Morning mood: Resting Heart Rate:

EXERCISE

CARDIO

Time and/or distance: Level: Heart Rate Max: Recovery:

STRENGTH: UPPER BODY & BACK		STRENGTH: LEGS & ABS	
1:	Reps:	1:	Reps:
2:	Reps:	2:	Reps:
3:	Reps:	3:	Reps:
4:	Reps:	4:	Reps:
5:	Reps:	5:	Reps:

FOOD

Breakfast:

Lunch:

Dinner:

Snacks: Crap: Booze:

LIFE

Caring, connecting, committing:

How did you do? ☐ Amazing ☐ Not Bad ☐ Shameful

Plans for tomorrow:

week 7

Exercise & Diet Plan for the Week

	MONDAY	TUESDAY	WEDNESDAY	THURSDAY	FRIDAY	SATURDAY	SUNDAY
CARDIO							
WEIGHTS							

Weight at beginning of week: _____ Weight at end of week: _____

Goals for the week:

Ideas for caring, connecting, committing:

HARRY SAYS: **PLAN YOUR FIRST KEDGE**

Our strong advice is to plan four kedging trips a year, because motivation and good intentions last three months—at most! So right now, even if it's cold and dark outside and you're feeling like a bear in hibernation, plan your first kedge. Perhaps a spring skiing trip or a hiking or biking tour with friends. It can be fancy or simple, expensive or dirt cheap, a weekend or a week, but a kedge should be hard for whatever shape you are in. And you should have your first one *written in stone* by the end of this week!

Monday | | |

How was your night? _____

Morning mood: _____ Resting Heart Rate: _____

EXERCISE

CARDIO

Time and/or distance: _____ Level: _____ Heart Rate Max: _____ Recovery: _____

STRENGTH: UPPER BODY & BACK		STRENGTH: LEGS & ABS	
1:	Reps:	1:	Reps:
2:	Reps:	2:	Reps:
3:	Reps:	3:	Reps:
4:	Reps:	4:	Reps:
5:	Reps:	5:	Reps:

FOOD

Breakfast:

Lunch:

Dinner:

Snacks: _____ Crap: _____ Booze: _____

LIFE

Caring, connecting, committing:

How did you do? ☐ Amazing ☐ Not Bad ☐ Shameful

Plans for tomorrow:

Tuesday ___ | | |

How was your night?	
Morning mood:	Resting Heart Rate:

E X E R C I S E

CARDIO

Time and/or distance: Level: Heart Rate Max: Recovery:

STRENGTH: UPPER BODY & BACK		STRENGTH: LEGS & ABS	
1:	Reps:	1:	Reps:
2:	Reps:	2:	Reps:
3:	Reps:	3:	Reps:
4:	Reps:	4:	Reps:
5:	Reps:	5:	Reps:

F O O D

Breakfast:

Lunch:

Dinner:

Snacks: Crap: Booze:

L I F E

Caring, connecting, committing:

How did you do? ☐ Amazing ☐ Not Bad ☐ Shameful

Plans for tomorrow:

Wednesday ___ | | |

How was your night?	
Morning mood:	Resting Heart Rate:

E X E R C I S E

CARDIO

Time and/or distance: Level: Heart Rate Max: Recovery:

STRENGTH: UPPER BODY & BACK		STRENGTH: LEGS & ABS	
1:	Reps:	1:	Reps:
2:	Reps:	2:	Reps:
3:	Reps:	3:	Reps:
4:	Reps:	4:	Reps:
5:	Reps:	5:	Reps:

F O O D

Breakfast:

Lunch:

Dinner:

Snacks: Crap: Booze:

L I F E

Caring, connecting, committing:

How did you do? ☐ Amazing ☐ Not Bad ☐ Shameful

Plans for tomorrow:

Thursday___|__|__|

How was your night?

Morning mood: Resting Heart Rate:

E X E R C I S E

CARDIO

Time and/or distance: Level: Heart Rate Max: Recovery:

STRENGTH: UPPER BODY & BACK		STRENGTH: LEGS & ABS	
1:	Reps:	1:	Reps:
2:	Reps:	2:	Reps:
3:	Reps:	3:	Reps:
4:	Reps:	4:	Reps:
5:	Reps:	5:	Reps:

F O O D

Breakfast:

Lunch:

Dinner:

Snacks: Crap: Booze:

L I F E

Caring, connecting, committing:

How did you do?   ☐ Amazing   ☐ Not Bad   ☐ Shameful

Plans for tomorrow:

Friday___|__|__|

How was your night?

Morning mood: Resting Heart Rate:

E X E R C I S E

CARDIO

Time and/or distance: Level: Heart Rate Max: Recovery:

STRENGTH: UPPER BODY & BACK		STRENGTH: LEGS & ABS	
1:	Reps:	1:	Reps:
2:	Reps:	2:	Reps:
3:	Reps:	3:	Reps:
4:	Reps:	4:	Reps:
5:	Reps:	5:	Reps:

F O O D

Breakfast:

Lunch:

Dinner:

Snacks: Crap: Booze:

L I F E

Caring, connecting, committing:

How did you do?   ☐ Amazing   ☐ Not Bad   ☐ Shameful

Plans for tomorrow:

Saturday ___ ___

How was your night?

Morning mood: Resting Heart Rate:

EXERCISE

CARDIO

Time and/or distance: Level: Heart Rate Max: Recovery:

STRENGTH: UPPER BODY & BACK		STRENGTH: LEGS & ABS	
1:	Reps:	1:	Reps:
2:	Reps:	2:	Reps:
3:	Reps:	3:	Reps:
4:	Reps:	4:	Reps:
5:	Reps:	5:	Reps:

FOOD

Breakfast:

Lunch:

Dinner:

Snacks: Crap: Booze:

LIFE

Caring, connecting, committing:

How did you do? ☐ Amazing ☐ Not Bad ☐ Shameful

Plans for tomorrow:

Sunday ___ ___

How was your night?

Morning mood: Resting Heart Rate:

EXERCISE

CARDIO

Time and/or distance: Level: Heart Rate Max: Recovery:

STRENGTH: UPPER BODY & BACK		STRENGTH: LEGS & ABS	
1:	Reps:	1:	Reps:
2:	Reps:	2:	Reps:
3:	Reps:	3:	Reps:
4:	Reps:	4:	Reps:
5:	Reps:	5:	Reps:

FOOD

Breakfast:

Lunch:

Dinner:

Snacks: Crap: Booze:

LIFE

Caring, connecting, committing:

How did you do? ☐ Amazing ☐ Not Bad ☐ Shameful

Plans for tomorrow:

8 week · Exercise & Diet Plan for the Week

	MONDAY	TUESDAY	WEDNESDAY	THURSDAY	FRIDAY	SATURDAY	SUNDAY
CARDIO							
WEIGHTS							

Weight at beginning of week: _____ Weight at end of week: _____

Goals for the week: _____

Ideas for caring, connecting, committing:

HARRY SAYS: DON'T WORRY ABOUT THE WEATHER

Go outdoors whenever possible. You can, you know, because there is no such thing as bad weather, only bad clothing choices. Seriously, spend fifteen minutes in your local outdoor store and you will be weatherproof for life. All it takes is a raincoat, rain pants, waterproof shoes, a rain hat and gloves, and you can walk or run year-round. The upside? The jogging path is less crowded when the weather's less than perfect. Besides, a long walk in the rain, cold, or snow is invigorating—as long as you're warm and dry.

Monday ___ | ___

How was your night? _____

Morning mood: _____ Resting Heart Rate: _____

EXERCISE

CARDIO

Time and/or distance: _____ Level: _____ Heart Rate Max: _____ Recovery: _____

STRENGTH: UPPER BODY & BACK		STRENGTH: LEGS & ABS	
1:	Reps:	1:	Reps:
2:	Reps:	2:	Reps:
3:	Reps:	3:	Reps:
4:	Reps:	4:	Reps:
5:	Reps:	5:	Reps:

FOOD

Breakfast:

Lunch:

Dinner:

Snacks: _____ Crap: _____ Booze: _____

LIFE

Caring, connecting, committing:

How did you do? ☐ Amazing ☐ Not Bad ☐ Shameful

Plans for tomorrow:

Tuesday _ | | |

How was your night?

Morning mood: Resting Heart Rate:

EXERCISE

CARDIO

Time and/or distance: Level: Heart Rate Max: Recovery:

STRENGTH: UPPER BODY & BACK		STRENGTH: LEGS & ABS	
1:	Reps:	1:	Reps:
2:	Reps:	2:	Reps:
3:	Reps:	3:	Reps:
4:	Reps:	4:	Reps:
5:	Reps:	5:	Reps:

FOOD

Breakfast:

Lunch:

Dinner:

Snacks: Crap: Booze:

LIFE

Caring, connecting, committing:

How did you do? ☐ Amazing ☐ Not Bad ☐ Shameful

Plans for tomorrow:

Wednesday _ | | |

How was your night?

Morning mood: Resting Heart Rate:

EXERCISE

CARDIO

Time and/or distance: Level: Heart Rate Max: Recovery:

STRENGTH: UPPER BODY & BACK		STRENGTH: LEGS & ABS	
1:	Reps:	1:	Reps:
2:	Reps:	2:	Reps:
3:	Reps:	3:	Reps:
4:	Reps:	4:	Reps:
5:	Reps:	5:	Reps:

FOOD

Breakfast:

Lunoh:

Dinner:

Snacks: Crap: Booze:

LIFE

Caring, connecting, committing:

How did you do? ☐ Amazing ☐ Not Bad ☐ Shameful

Plans for tomorrow:

Thursday ___ | ___ | ___ |

How was your night?

Morning mood: Resting Heart Rate:

CARDIO

Time and/or distance: Level: Heart Rate Max: Recovery:

STRENGTH: UPPER BODY & BACK		STRENGTH: LEGS & ABS	
1:	Reps:	1:	Reps:
2:	Reps:	2:	Reps:
3:	Reps:	3:	Reps:
4:	Reps:	4:	Reps:
5:	Reps:	5:	Reps:

Breakfast:

Lunch:

Dinner:

Snacks: Crap: Booze:

Caring, connecting, committing:

How did you do? ☐ Amazing ☐ Not Bad ☐ Shameful

Plans for tomorrow:

Friday ___ | ___ | ___ |

How was your night?

Morning mood: Resting Heart Rate:

CARDIO

Time and/or distance: Level: Heart Rate Max: Recovery:

STRENGTH: UPPER BODY & BACK		STRENGTH: LEGS & ABS	
1:	Reps:	1:	Reps:
2:	Reps:	2:	Reps:
3:	Reps:	3:	Reps:
4:	Reps:	4:	Reps:
5:	Reps:	5:	Reps:

Breakfast:

Lunch:

Dinner:

Snacks: Crap: Booze:

Caring, connecting, committing:

How did you do? ☐ Amazing ☐ Not Bad ☐ Shameful

Plans for tomorrow:

Saturday___|___|___

How was your night?

Morning mood: Resting Heart Rate:

EXERCISE

CARDIO

Time and/or distance: Level: Heart Rate Max: Recovery:

STRENGTH: UPPER BODY & BACK		STRENGTH: LEGS & ABS	
1:	Reps:	1:	Reps:
2:	Reps:	2:	Reps:
3:	Reps:	3:	Reps:
4:	Reps:	4:	Reps:
5:	Reps:	5:	Reps:

FOOD

Breakfast:

Lunch:

Dinner:

Snacks: Crap: Booze:

LIFE

Caring, connecting, committing:

How did you do?   ☐ Amazing ☐ Not Bad ☐ Shameful

Plans for tomorrow:

Sunday___|___|___

How was your night?

Morning mood: Resting Heart Rate:

EXERCISE

CARDIO

Time and/or distance: Level: Heart Rate Max: Recovery:

STRENGTH: UPPER BODY & BACK		STRENGTH: LEGS & ABS	
1:	Reps:	1:	Reps:
2:	Reps:	2:	Reps:
3:	Reps:	3:	Reps:
4:	Reps:	4:	Reps:
5:	Reps:	5:	Reps:

FOOD

Breakfast:

Lunch:

Dinner:

Snacks: Crap: Booze:

LIFE

Caring, connecting, committing:

How did you do?   ☐ Amazing ☐ Not Bad ☐ Shameful

Plans for tomorrow:

9 week

Exercise & Diet Plan for the Week

	MONDAY	TUESDAY	WEDNESDAY	THURSDAY	FRIDAY	SATURDAY	SUNDAY
CARDIO							
WEIGHTS							

Weight at beginning of week: _____ Weight at end of week: _____

Goals for the week: _____

Ideas for caring, connecting, committing: _____

CHRIS SAYS: DO WEIGHTS!

Have you hired a trainer yet? Do it. In fact, do *anything* that helps you keep up with the weights. The hardest part of the exercise regimen, for most, is weight training. Well, do it anyway. Weight training is the antidote to sore joints (*the* great curse of old age), and it does wonders for balance. Bottom line: Weight training isn't about muscles so much as it's about the quality of your life . . . now and in the future.

Monday | | |

How was your night?

Morning mood: _____ **Resting Heart Rate:** _____

EXERCISE

CARDIO

Time and/or distance: _____ Level: _____ Heart Rate Max: _____ Recovery: _____

STRENGTH: UPPER BODY & BACK		STRENGTH: LEGS & ABS	
1:	Reps:	1:	Reps:
2:	Reps:	2:	Reps:
3:	Reps:	3:	Reps:
4:	Reps:	4:	Reps:
5:	Reps:	5:	Reps:

FOOD

Breakfast:

Lunch:

Dinner:

Snacks: _____ Crap: _____ Booze: _____

LIFE

Caring, connecting, committing:

How did you do? ☐ Amazing ☐ Not Bad ☐ Shameful

Plans for tomorrow:

Tuesday _ | | |

How was your night?

Morning mood: Resting Heart Rate:

E X E R C I S E

CARDIO

Time and/or distance: Level: Heart Rate Max: Recovery:

STRENGTH: UPPER BODY & BACK		STRENGTH: LEGS & ABS	
1:	Reps:	1:	Reps:
2:	Reps:	2:	Reps:
3:	Reps:	3:	Reps:
4:	Reps:	4:	Reps:
5:	Reps:	5:	Reps:

F O O D

Breakfast:

Lunch:

Dinner:

Snacks: Crap: Booze:

L I F E

Caring, connecting, committing.

How did you do?   ☐ Amazing ☐ Not Bad ☐ Shameful

Plans for tomorrow:

Wednesday _ | | |

How was your night?

Morning mood: Resting Heart Rate:

E X E R C I S E

CARDIO

Time and/or distance: Level: Heart Rate Max: Recovery:

STRENGTH: UPPER BODY & BACK		STRENGTH: LEGS & ABS	
1:	Reps:	1:	Reps:
2:	Reps:	2:	Reps:
3:	Reps:	3:	Reps:
4:	Reps:	4:	Reps:
5:	Reps:	5:	Reps:

F O O D

Breakfast:

Lunch:

Dinner:

Snacks: Crap: Booze:

L I F E

Caring, connecting, committing:

How did you do?   ☐ Amazing ☐ Not Bad ☐ Shameful

Plans for tomorrow:

Thursday ⎿ ⎿ ⎿

How was your night?

Morning mood: Resting Heart Rate:

EXERCISE

CARDIO

Time and/or distance: Level: Heart Rate Max: Recovery:

STRENGTH: UPPER BODY & BACK		STRENGTH: LEGS & ABS	
1:	Reps:	1:	Reps:
2:	Reps:	2:	Reps:
3:	Reps:	3:	Reps:
4:	Reps:	4:	Reps:
5:	Reps:	5:	Reps:

FOOD

Breakfast:

Lunch:

Dinner:

Snacks: Crap: Booze:

LIFE

Caring, connecting, committing:

How did you do?   ☐ Amazing   ☐ Not Bad   ☐ Shameful

Plans for tomorrow:

Friday ⎿ ⎿ ⎿

How was your night?

Morning mood: Resting Heart Rate:

EXERCISE

CARDIO

Time and/or distance: Level: Heart Rate Max: Recovery:

STRENGTH: UPPER BODY & BACK		STRENGTH: LEGS & ABS	
1:	Reps:	1:	Reps:
2:	Reps:	2:	Reps:
3:	Reps:	3:	Reps:
4:	Reps:	4:	Reps:
5:	Reps:	5:	Reps:

FOOD

Breakfast:

Lunch:

Dinner:

Snacks: Crap: Booze:

LIFE

Caring, connecting, committing:

How did you do?   ☐ Amazing   ☐ Not Bad   ☐ Shameful

Plans for tomorrow:

Saturday___|___|___|

How was your night?	
Morning mood:	Resting Heart Rate:

E X E R C I S E

CARDIO

Time and/or distance:	Level:	Heart Rate Max:	Recovery:

STRENGTH: UPPER BODY & BACK		STRENGTH: LEGS & ABS	
1:	Reps:	1:	Reps:
2:	Reps:	2:	Reps:
3:	Reps:	3:	Reps:
4:	Reps:	4:	Reps:
5:	Reps:	5:	Reps:

F O O D

Breakfast:

Lunch:

Dinner:

Snacks:	Crap:	Booze:

L I F E

Caring, connecting, committing:

How did you do? ☐ Amazing ☐ Not Bad ☐ Shameful

Plans for tomorrow:

Sunday___|___|___|

How was your night?	
Morning mood:	Resting Heart Rate:

E X E R C I S E

CARDIO

Time and/or distance:	Level:	Heart Rate Max:	Recovery:

STRENGTH: UPPER BODY & BACK		STRENGTH: LEGS & ABS	
1:	Reps:	1:	Reps:
2:	Reps:	2:	Reps:
3:	Reps:	3:	Reps:
4:	Reps:	4:	Reps:
5:	Reps:	5:	Reps:

F O O D

Breakfast:

Lunch:

Dinner:

Snacks:	Crap:	Booze:

L I F E

Caring, connecting, committing:

How did you do? ☐ Amazing ☐ Not Bad ☐ Shameful

Plans for tomorrow:

Exercise & Diet Plan for the Week

	MONDAY	TUESDAY	WEDNESDAY	THURSDAY	FRIDAY	SATURDAY	SUNDAY
CARDIO							
WEIGHTS							

Weight at beginning of week: Weight at end of week:

Goals for the week:

Ideas for caring, connecting, committing:

HARRY SAYS: DON'T THINK YOU CAN WALK ON YOUR HANDS

Strength training *is* the great key to feeling healthy in the Next Third, and you really should do it at least two days and maybe three a week. Do all the parts of your body . . . upper body, lower, and core. But if things get tough, never fail to lift weights with your legs and work to make them strong. Strong legs save you from falls and keep you young. When in doubt, default to leg exercises. They are what will keep you off the walker and out of the wheelchair. You can't walk on your hands.

Monday ___ | | |

How was your night?

Morning mood: Resting Heart Rate:

EXERCISE

CARDIO

Time and/or distance: Level: Heart Rate Max: Recovery:

STRENGTH: UPPER BODY & BACK		STRENGTH: LEGS & ABS	
1:	Reps:	1:	Reps:
2:	Reps:	2:	Reps:
3:	Reps:	3:	Reps:
4:	Reps:	4:	Reps:
5:	Reps:	5:	Reps:

FOOD

Breakfast:

Lunch:

Dinner:

Snacks: Crap: Booze:

LIFE

Caring, connecting, committing:

How did you do? ☐ Amazing ☐ Not Bad ☐ Shameful

Plans for tomorrow:

Tuesday___ | | |

How was your night?	
Morning mood:	Resting Heart Rate:

EXERCISE

CARDIO

Time and/or distance:	Level:	Heart Rate Max:	Recovery:

STRENGTH: UPPER BODY & BACK		STRENGTH: LEGS & ABS	
1:	Reps:	1:	Reps:
2:	Reps:	2:	Reps:
3:	Reps:	3:	Reps:
4:	Reps:	4:	Reps:
5:	Reps:	5:	Reps:

FOOD

Breakfast:

Lunch:

Dinner:

Snacks:	Crap:	Booze:

LIFE

Caring, connecting, committing:

How did you do?   ☐ Amazing   ☐ Not Bad   ☐ Shameful

Plans for tomorrow:

Wednesday___ | | |

How was your night?	
Morning mood:	Resting Heart Rate:

EXERCISE

CARDIO

Time and/or distance:	Level:	Heart Rate Max:	Recovery:

STRENGTH: UPPER BODY & BACK		STRENGTH: LEGS & ABS	
1:	Reps:	1:	Reps:
2:	Reps:	2:	Reps:
3:	Reps:	3:	Reps:
4:	Reps:	4:	Reps:
5:	Reps:	5:	Reps:

FOOD

Breakfast:

Lunch:

Dinner:

Snacks:	Crap:	Booze:

LIFE

Caring, connecting, committing:

How did you do?   ☐ Amazing   ☐ Not Bad   ☐ Shameful

Plans for tomorrow:

Thursday ___ | | |

How was your night?

Morning mood: Resting Heart Rate:

E X E R C I S E

CARDIO

Time and/or distance:	Level:	Heart Rate Max:	Recovery:

STRENGTH: UPPER BODY & BACK		STRENGTH: LEGS & ABS	
1:	Reps:	1:	Reps:
2:	Reps:	2:	Reps:
3:	Reps:	3:	Reps:
4:	Reps:	4:	Reps:
5:	Reps:	5:	Reps:

F O O D

Breakfast:

Lunch:

Dinner:

Snacks:	Crap:	Booze:

L I F E

Caring, connecting, committing:

How did you do?   ☐ Amazing   ☐ Not Bad   ☐ Shameful

Plans for tomorrow:

Friday ___ | | |

How was your night?

Morning mood: Resting Heart Rate:

E X E R C I S E

CARDIO

Time and/or distance:	Level:	Heart Rate Max:	Recovery:

STRENGTH: UPPER BODY & BACK		STRENGTH: LEGS & ABS	
1:	Reps:	1:	Reps:
2:	Reps:	2:	Reps:
3:	Reps:	3:	Reps:
4:	Reps:	4:	Reps:
5:	Reps:	5:	Reps:

F O O D

Breakfast:

Lunch:

Dinner:

Snacks:	Crap:	Booze:

L I F E

Caring, connecting, committing:

How did you do?   ☐ Amazing   ☐ Not Bad   ☐ Shameful

Plans for tomorrow:

Saturday _ | | |

How was your night?

Morning mood: Resting Heart Rate:

E X E R C I S E

CARDIO

Time and/or distance: Level: Heart Rate Max: Recovery:

STRENGTH: UPPER BODY & BACK		STRENGTH: LEGS & ABS	
1:	Reps:	1:	Reps:
2:	Reps:	2:	Reps:
3:	Reps:	3:	Reps:
4:	Reps:	4:	Reps:
5:	Reps:	5:	Reps:

F O O D

Breakfast:

Lunch:

Dinner:

Snacks: Crap: Booze:

L I F E

Caring, connecting, committing:

How did you do?   ☐ Amazing   ☐ Not Bad   ☐ Shameful

Plans for tomorrow:

Sunday _ | | |

How was your night?

Morning mood: Resting Heart Rate:

E X E R C I S E

CARDIO

Time and/or distance: Level: Heart Rate Max: Recovery:

STRENGTH: UPPER BODY & BACK		STRENGTH: LEGS & ABS	
1:	Reps:	1:	Reps:
2:	Reps:	2:	Reps:
3:	Reps:	3:	Reps:
4:	Reps:	4:	Reps:
5:	Reps:	5:	Reps:

F O O D

Breakfast:

Lunch:

Dinner:

Snacks: Crap: Booze:

L I F E

Caring, connecting, committing:

How did you do?   ☐ Amazing   ☐ Not Bad   ☐ Shameful

Plans for tomorrow:

11
week

Exercise & Diet Plan for the Week

	MONDAY	TUESDAY	WEDNESDAY	THURSDAY	FRIDAY	SATURDAY	SUNDAY
CARDIO							
WEIGHTS							

Weight at beginning of week: _____ Weight at end of week: _____

Goals for the week: _____

Ideas for caring, connecting, committing: _____

CHRIS SAYS: TRY THE YOGA SUBSTITUTE

If you absolutely detest weight training, you might try yoga. Serious yoga, with lots of "downward dogs" and other hard poses, is a kind of substitute for weight training for some. And it's sensational for your balance. Some say it can be a substitute for aerobics, too, but we're skeptical about that. Best stay with some flat-out aerobics to go with the yoga.

Monday ___ | ___ |

How was your night?

Morning mood: _____ Resting Heart Rate: _____

EXERCISE

CARDIO

Time and/or distance: _____ Level: _____ Heart Rate Max: _____ Recovery: _____

STRENGTH: UPPER BODY & BACK		STRENGTH: LEGS & ABS	
1:	Reps:	1:	Reps:
2:	Reps:	2:	Reps:
3:	Reps:	3:	Reps:
4:	Reps:	4:	Reps:
5:	Reps:	5:	Reps:

FOOD

Breakfast:

Lunch:

Dinner:

Snacks: _____ Crap: _____ Booze: _____

LIFE

Caring, connecting, committing:

How did you do? ☐ Amazing ☐ Not Bad ☐ Shameful

Plans for tomorrow:

Tuesday___ | | |

How was your night?

Morning mood: Resting Heart Rate:

EXERCISE

CARDIO

Time and/or distance: Level: Heart Rate Max: Recovery:

STRENGTH: UPPER BODY & BACK		STRENGTH: LEGS & ABS	
1:	Reps:	1:	Reps:
2:	Reps:	2:	Reps:
3:	Reps:	3:	Reps:
4:	Reps:	4:	Reps:
5:	Reps:	5:	Reps:

FOOD

Breakfast:

Lunch:

Dinner:

Snacks: Crap: Booze:

LIFE

Caring, connecting, committing:

How did you do?   ☐ Amazing   ☐ Not Bad   ☐ Shameful

Plans for tomorrow:

Wednesday___ | | |

How was your night?

Morning mood: Resting Heart Rate:

EXERCISE

CARDIO

Time and/or distance: Level: Heart Rate Max: Recovery:

STRENGTH: UPPER BODY & BACK		STRENGTH: LEGS & ABS	
1:	Reps:	1:	Reps:
2:	Reps:	2:	Reps:
3:	Reps:	3:	Reps:
4:	Reps:	4:	Reps:
5:	Reps:	5:	Reps:

FOOD

Breakfast:

Lunch:

Dinner:

Snacks: Crap: Booze:

LIFE

Caring, connecting, committing:

How did you do?   ☐ Amazing   ☐ Not Bad   ☐ Shameful

Plans for tomorrow:

Thursday___|__|__|

How was your night?

Morning mood: Resting Heart Rate:

E X E R C I S E

CARDIO

Time and/or distance: Level: Heart Rate Max: Recovery:

STRENGTH: UPPER BODY & BACK		STRENGTH: LEGS & ABS	
1:	Reps:	1:	Reps:
2:	Reps:	2:	Reps:
3:	Reps:	3:	Reps:
4:	Reps:	4:	Reps:
5:	Reps:	5:	Reps:

F O O D

Breakfast:

Lunch:

Dinner:

Snacks: Crap: Booze:

L I F E

Caring, connecting, committing:

How did you do?   ☐ Amazing ☐ Not Bad ☐ Shameful

Plans for tomorrow:

Friday___|__|__|

How was your night?

Morning mood: Resting Heart Rate:

E X E R C I S E

CARDIO

Time and/or distance: Level: Heart Rate Max: Recovery:

STRENGTH: UPPER BODY & BACK		STRENGTH: LEGS & ABS	
1:	Reps:	1:	Reps:
2:	Reps:	2:	Reps:
3:	Reps:	3:	Reps:
4:	Reps:	4:	Reps:
5:	Reps:	5:	Reps:

F O O D

Breakfast:

Lunch:

Dinner:

Snacks: Crap: Booze:

L I F E

Caring, connecting, committing:

How did you do?   ☐ Amazing ☐ Not Bad ☐ Shameful

Plans for tomorrow:

Saturday___|__|__|

How was your night?

Morning mood: Resting Heart Rate:

E X E R C I S E

CARDIO

Time and/or distance: Level: Heart Rate Max: Recovery:

STRENGTH: UPPER BODY & BACK		**STRENGTH: LEGS & ABS**	
1:	Reps:	1:	Reps:
2:	Reps:	2:	Reps:
3:	Reps:	3:	Reps:
4:	Reps:	4:	Reps:
5:	Reps:	5:	Reps:

F O O D

Breakfast:

Lunch:

Dinner:

Snacks: Crap: Booze:

L I F E

Caring, connecting, committing:

How did you do?   ☐ Amazing   ☐ Not Bad   ☐ Shameful

Plans for tomorrow:

Sunday___|__|__|

How was your night?

Morning mood: Resting Heart Rate:

E X E R C I S E

CARDIO

Time and/or distance: Level: Heart Rate Max: Recovery:

STRENGTH: UPPER BODY & BACK		**STRENGTH: LEGS & ABS**	
1:	Reps:	1:	Reps:
2:	Reps:	2:	Reps:
3:	Reps:	3:	Reps:
4:	Reps:	4:	Reps:
5:	Reps:	5:	Reps:

F O O D

Breakfast:

Lunch:

Dinner:

Snacks: Crap: Booze:

L I F E

Caring, connecting, committing:

How did you do?   ☐ Amazing   ☐ Not Bad   ☐ Shameful

Plans for tomorrow:

Exercise & Diet Plan for the Week

	MONDAY	TUESDAY	WEDNESDAY	THURSDAY	FRIDAY	SATURDAY	SUNDAY
CARDIO							
WEIGHTS							

Weight at beginning of week: Weight at end of week:

Goals for the week:

Ideas for caring, connecting, committing:

HARRY SAYS: FIGHT ROT AT THE CORE

Default to legs if you must, but it is also terribly important to strengthen your core . . . in other words, your torso or trunk. That means abdominals, of course, but also the whole wrap of muscles surrounding your trunk—the front, sides, and back. Ask your trainer for some tips. Or you may want to try Pilates, which is heavily focused on core and which some people love.

Monday_ | | |

How was your night?

Morning mood: Resting Heart Rate:

E X E R C I S E

CARDIO

Time and/or distance: Level: Heart Rate Max: Recovery:

STRENGTH: UPPER BODY & BACK		**STRENGTH: LEGS & ABS**	
1:	Reps:	1:	Reps:
2:	Reps:	2:	Reps:
3:	Reps:	3:	Reps:
4:	Reps:	4:	Reps:
5:	Reps:	5:	Reps:

F O O D

Breakfast:

Lunch:

Dinner:

Snacks: Crap: Booze:

L I F E

Caring, connecting, committing:

How did you do?   ☐ Amazing   ☐ Not Bad   ☐ Shameful

Plans for tomorrow:

Tuesday___ | | |

How was your night?

Morning mood: Resting Heart Rate:

EXERCISE

CARDIO

Time and/or distance: Level: Heart Rate Max: Recovery:

STRENGTH: UPPER BODY & BACK		STRENGTH: LEGS & ABS	
1:	Reps:	1:	Reps:
2:	Reps:	2:	Reps:
3:	Reps:	3:	Reps:
4:	Reps:	4:	Reps:
5:	Reps:	5:	Reps:

FOOD

Breakfast:

Lunch:

Dinner:

Snacks: Crap: Booze:

LIFE

Caring, connecting, committing:

How did you do?   ☐ Amazing   ☐ Not Bad   ☐ Shameful

Plans for tomorrow:

Wednesday___ | | |

How was your night?

Morning mood: Resting Heart Rate:

EXERCISE

CARDIO

Time and/or distance: Level: Heart Rate Max: Recovery:

STRENGTH: UPPER BODY & BACK		STRENGTH: LEGS & ABS	
1:	Reps:	1:	Reps:
2:	Reps:	2:	Reps:
3:	Reps:	3:	Reps:
4:	Reps:	4:	Reps:
5:	Reps:	5:	Reps:

FOOD

Breakfast:

Lunch:

Dinner:

Snacks: Crap: Booze:

LIFE

Caring, connecting, committing:

How did you do?   ☐ Amazing   ☐ Not Bad   ☐ Shameful

Plans for tomorrow:

Thursday____|__|__|

How was your night?

Morning mood: Resting Heart Rate:

E X E R C I S E

CARDIO

Time and/or distance: Level: Heart Rate Max: Recovery:

STRENGTH: UPPER BODY & BACK		**STRENGTH: LEGS & ABS**	
1:	Reps:	1:	Reps:
2:	Reps:	2:	Reps:
3:	Reps:	3:	Reps:
4:	Reps:	4:	Reps:
5:	Reps:	5:	Reps:

F O O D

Breakfast:

Lunch:

Dinner:

Snacks: Crap: Booze:

L I F E

Caring, connecting, committing:

How did you do?   ☐ Amazing ☐ Not Bad ☐ Shameful

Plans for tomorrow:

Friday____|__|__|

How was your night?

Morning mood: Resting Heart Rate:

E X E R C I S E

CARDIO

Time and/or distance: Level: Heart Rate Max: Recovery:

STRENGTH: UPPER BODY & BACK		**STRENGTH: LEGS & ABS**	
1:	Reps:	1:	Reps:
2:	Reps:	2:	Reps:
3:	Reps:	3:	Reps:
4:	Reps:	4:	Reps:
5:	Reps:	5:	Reps:

F O O D

Breakfast:

Lunch:

Dinner:

Snacks: Crap: Booze:

L I F E

Caring, connecting, committing:

How did you do?   ☐ Amazing ☐ Not Bad ☐ Shameful

Plans for tomorrow:

Saturday___|__|__|

How was your night?

Morning mood: Resting Heart Rate:

EXERCISE

CARDIO

Time and/or distance: Level: Heart Rate Max: Recovery:

STRENGTH: UPPER BODY & BACK		STRENGTH: LEGS & ABS	
1:	Reps:	1:	Reps:
2:	Reps:	2:	Reps:
3:	Reps:	3:	Reps:
4:	Reps:	4:	Reps:
5:	Reps:	5:	Reps:

FOOD

Breakfast:

Lunch:

Dinner:

Snacks: Crap: Booze:

LIFE

Caring, connecting, committing:

How did you do? ☐ Amazing ☐ Not Bad ☐ Shameful

Plans for tomorrow:

Sunday___|__|__|

How was your night?

Morning mood: Resting Heart Rate:

EXERCISE

CARDIO

Time and/or distance: Level: Heart Rate Max: Recovery:

STRENGTH: UPPER BODY & BACK		STRENGTH: LEGS & ABS	
1:	Reps:	1:	Reps:
2:	Reps:	2:	Reps:
3:	Reps:	3:	Reps:
4:	Reps:	4:	Reps:
5:	Reps:	5:	Reps:

FOOD

Breakfast:

Lunch:

Dinner:

Snacks: Crap: Booze:

LIFE

Caring, connecting, committing:

How did you do? ☐ Amazing ☐ Not Bad ☐ Shameful

Plans for tomorrow:

Exercise & Diet Plan for the Week

	MONDAY	TUESDAY	WEDNESDAY	THURSDAY	FRIDAY	SATURDAY	SUNDAY
CARDIO							
WEIGHTS							

Weight at beginning of week: Weight at end of week:

Goals for the week:

Ideas for caring, connecting, committing:

HARRY SAYS: **PLAN YOUR SECOND KEDGE**

By now you should have finished your first kedge—reinvigorated your commitment, tested yourself, and ended up feeling pretty good about yourself. Or maybe you didn't get around to it; either way, the clock starts again! Warm-weather climates offer the most kedging options—tennis camps, bike trips, canoe trips, mini-triathlons, 5K and 10K road races . . . the list goes on for miles. Planning for a Fourth of July (or Caribbean!) kedge will pull you along with a surge of energy and enthusiasm. Make your plan this week. Try to get some friends to join, but even if it's just you, GET YOUNGER!

Monday | | |

How was your night?

Morning mood: Resting Heart Rate:

E X E R C I S E

CARDIO

Time and/or distance: Level: Heart Rate Max: Recovery:

STRENGTH: UPPER BODY & BACK		STRENGTH: LEGS & ABS	
1:	Reps:	1:	Reps:
2:	Reps:	2:	Reps:
3:	Reps:	3:	Reps:
4:	Reps:	4:	Reps:
5:	Reps:	5:	Reps:

F O O D

Breakfast:

Lunch:

Dinner:

Snacks: Crap: Booze:

L I F E

Caring, connecting, committing:

How did you do? ☐ Amazing ☐ Not Bad ☐ Shameful

Plans for tomorrow:

Tuesday _|_|_

How was your night?

Morning mood: Resting Heart Rate:

E X E R C I S E

CARDIO

Time and/or distance: Level: Heart Rate Max: Recovery:

STRENGTH: UPPER BODY & BACK		STRENGTH: LEGS & ABS	
1:	Reps:	1:	Reps:
2:	Reps:	2:	Reps:
3:	Reps:	3:	Reps:
4:	Reps:	4:	Reps:
5:	Reps:	5:	Reps:

F O O D

Breakfast:

Lunch:

Dinner:

Snacks: Crap: Booze:

L I F E

Caring, connecting, committing:

How did you do?   ☐ Amazing   ☐ Not Bad   ☐ Shameful

Plans for tomorrow:

Wednesday _|_|_

How was your night?

Morning mood: Resting Heart Rate:

E X E R C I S E

CARDIO

Time and/or distance: Level: Heart Rate Max: Recovery:

STRENGTH: UPPER BODY & BACK		STRENGTH: LEGS & ABS	
1:	Reps:	1:	Reps:
2:	Reps:	2:	Reps:
3:	Reps:	3:	Reps.
4:	Reps:	4:	Reps:
5:	Reps:	5:	Reps:

F O O D

Breakfast:

Lunch:

Dinner:

Snacks: Crap: Booze:

L I F E

Caring, connecting, committing:

How did you do?   ☐ Amazing   ☐ Not Bad   ☐ Shameful

Plans for tomorrow:

Thursday___ | | |

How was your night?

Morning mood: Resting Heart Rate:

E X E R C I S E

CARDIO

Time and/or distance: Level: Heart Rate Max: Recovery:

STRENGTH: UPPER BODY & BACK		**STRENGTH: LEGS & ABS**	
1:	Reps:	1:	Reps:
2:	Reps:	2:	Reps:
3:	Reps:	3:	Reps:
4:	Reps:	4:	Reps:
5:	Reps:	5:	Reps:

F O O D

Breakfast:

Lunch:

Dinner:

Snacks: Crap: Booze:

L I F E

Caring, connecting, committing:

How did you do?   ☐ Amazing ☐ Not Bad ☐ Shameful

Plans for tomorrow:

Friday___ | | |

How was your night?

Morning mood: Resting Heart Rate:

E X E R C I S E

CARDIO

Time and/or distance: Level: Heart Rate Max: Recovery:

STRENGTH: UPPER BODY & BACK		**STRENGTH: LEGS & ABS**	
1:	Reps:	1:	Reps:
2:	Reps:	2:	Reps:
3:	Reps:	3:	Reps:
4:	Reps:	4:	Reps:
5:	Reps:	5:	Reps:

F O O D

Breakfast:

Lunch:

Dinner:

Snacks: Crap: Booze:

L I F E

Caring, connecting, committing:

How did you do?   ☐ Amazing ☐ Not Bad ☐ Shameful

Plans for tomorrow:

Saturday ___ | | |

How was your night?

Morning mood: Resting Heart Rate:

EXERCISE

CARDIO

Time and/or distance: Level: Heart Rate Max: Recovery:

STRENGTH: UPPER BODY & BACK		STRENGTH: LEGS & ABS	
1:	Reps:	1:	Reps:
2:	Reps:	2:	Reps:
3:	Reps:	3:	Reps:
4:	Reps:	4:	Reps:
5:	Reps:	5:	Reps:

FOOD

Breakfast:

Lunch:

Dinner:

Snacks: Crap: Booze:

LIFE

Caring, connecting, committing:

How did you do?   ☐ Amazing   ☐ Not Bad   ☐ Shameful

Plans for tomorrow:

Sunday ___ | | |

How was your night?

Morning mood: Resting Heart Rate:

EXERCISE

CARDIO

Time and/or distance: Level: Heart Rate Max: Recovery:

STRENGTH: UPPER BODY & BACK		STRENGTH: LEGS & ABS	
1:	Reps:	1:	Reps:
2:	Reps:	2:	Reps:
3:	Reps:	3:	Reps:
4:	Reps:	4:	Reps:
5:	Reps:	5:	Reps:

FOOD

Breakfast:

Lunch:

Dinner:

Snacks: Crap: Booze:

LIFE

Caring, connecting, committing:

How did you do?   ☐ Amazing   ☐ Not Bad   ☐ Shameful

Plans for tomorrow:

Exercise & Diet Plan for the Week

	MONDAY	TUESDAY	WEDNESDAY	THURSDAY	FRIDAY	SATURDAY	SUNDAY
CARDIO							
WEIGHTS							

Weight at beginning of week: _____ Weight at end of week: _____

Goals for the week:

Ideas for caring, connecting, committing:

CHRIS SAYS: **TAKE A CLASS**

Spinning classes are my craziness, but anything that gets you to the gym regularly is fine. Try dance, yoga . . . it doesn't matter. It's so much easier to get to the gym if there is a regular class. And once you're there, the class keeps you going. That dreadful music . . . the shouts of the teenage instructor . . . it all works. We're mammals; we do better in groups.

Monday ___ | | |

How was your night? _____

Morning mood: _____ Resting Heart Rate: _____

E X E R C I S E

CARDIO

Time and/or distance: _____ Level: _____ Heart Rate Max: _____ Recovery: _____

STRENGTH: UPPER BODY & BACK		**STRENGTH: LEGS & ABS**	
1:	Reps:	1:	Reps:
2:	Reps:	2:	Reps:
3:	Reps:	3:	Reps:
4:	Reps:	4:	Reps:
5:	Reps:	5:	Reps:

F O O D

Breakfast:

Lunch:

Dinner:

Snacks: _____ Crap: _____ Booze: _____

L I F E

Caring, connecting, committing:

How did you do? ☐ Amazing ☐ Not Bad ☐ Shameful

Plans for tomorrow:

Tuesday____|__|__|

How was your night?

Morning mood: Resting Heart Rate:

E X E R C I S E

CARDIO

Time and/or distance: Level: Heart Rate Max: Recovery:

STRENGTH: UPPER BODY & BACK		STRENGTH: LEGS & ABS	
1:	Reps:	1:	Reps:
2:	Reps:	2:	Reps:
3:	Reps:	3:	Reps:
4:	Reps:	4:	Reps:
5:	Reps:	5:	Reps:

F O O D

Breakfast:

Lunch:

Dinner:

Snacks: Crap: Booze:

L I F E

Caring, connecting, committing:

How did you do?   ☐ Amazing ☐ Not Bad ☐ Shameful

Plans for tomorrow:

Wednesday____|__|__|

How was your night?

Morning mood: Resting Heart Rate:

E X E R C I S E

CARDIO

Time and/or distance: Level: Heart Rate Max: Recovery:

STRENGTH: UPPER BODY & BACK		STRENGTH: LEGS & ABS	
1:	Reps:	1:	Reps:
2:	Reps:	2:	Reps:
3:	Reps:	3:	Reps:
4:	Reps:	4:	Reps:
5:	Reps:	5:	Reps:

F O O D

Breakfast:

Lunch:

Dinner:

Snacks: Crap: Booze:

L I F E

Caring, connecting, committing:

How did you do?   ☐ Amazing ☐ Not Bad ☐ Shameful

Plans for tomorrow:

Thursday␣␣|␣␣|␣␣|

How was your night?

Morning mood:␣␣␣␣␣␣Resting Heart Rate:

E X E R C I S E

CARDIO

Time and/or distance:␣␣␣␣Level:␣␣␣␣Heart Rate Max:␣␣␣␣Recovery:

STRENGTH: UPPER BODY & BACK		STRENGTH: LEGS & ABS	
1:	Reps:	1:	Reps:
2:	Reps:	2:	Reps:
3:	Reps:	3:	Reps:
4:	Reps:	4:	Reps:
5:	Reps:	5:	Reps:

F O O D

Breakfast:

Lunch:

Dinner:

Snacks:␣␣␣␣␣␣Crap:␣␣␣␣␣␣Booze:

L I F E

Caring, connecting, committing:

How did you do?␣␣☐ Amazing␣␣☐ Not Bad␣␣☐ Shameful

Plans for tomorrow:

Friday␣␣|␣␣|␣␣|

How was your night?

Morning mood:␣␣␣␣␣␣Resting Heart Rate:

E X E R C I S E

CARDIO

Time and/or distance:␣␣␣␣Level:␣␣␣␣Heart Rate Max:␣␣␣␣Recovery:

STRENGTH: UPPER BODY & BACK		STRENGTH: LEGS & ABS	
1:	Reps:	1:	Reps:
2:	Reps:	2:	Reps:
3:	Reps:	3:	Reps:
4:	Reps:	4:	Reps:
5:	Reps:	5:	Reps:

F O O D

Breakfast:

Lunch:

Dinner:

Snacks:␣␣␣␣␣␣Crap:␣␣␣␣␣␣Booze:

L I F E

Caring, connecting, committing:

How did you do?␣␣☐ Amazing␣␣☐ Not Bad␣␣☐ Shameful

Plans for tomorrow:

Saturday ___ | | |

How was your night?

Morning mood: Resting Heart Rate:

E X E R C I S E

CARDIO

Time and/or distance: Level: Heart Rate Max: Recovery:

STRENGTH: UPPER BODY & BACK		**STRENGTH: LEGS & ABS**	
1:	Reps:	1:	Reps:
2:	Reps:	2:	Reps:
3:	Reps:	3:	Reps:
4:	Reps:	4:	Reps:
5:	Reps:	5:	Reps:

F O O D

Breakfast:

Lunch:

Dinner:

Snacks: Crap: Booze:

L I F E

Caring, connecting, committing:

How did you do?   ☐ Amazing   ☐ Not Bad   ☐ Shameful

Plans for tomorrow:

Sunday ___ | | |

How was your night?

Morning mood: Resting Heart Rate:

E X E R C I S E

CARDIO

Time and/or distance: Level: Heart Rate Max: Recovery:

STRENGTH: UPPER BODY & BACK		**STRENGTH: LEGS & ABS**	
1:	Reps:	1:	Reps:
2:	Reps:	2:	Reps:
3:	Reps:	3:	Reps:
4:	Reps:	4:	Reps:
5:	Reps:	5:	Reps:

F O O D

Breakfast:

Lunch:

Dinner:

Snacks: Crap: Booze:

L I F E

Caring, connecting, committing:

How did you do?   ☐ Amazing   ☐ Not Bad   ☐ Shameful

Plans for tomorrow:

Exercise & Diet Plan for the Week

	MONDAY	TUESDAY	WEDNESDAY	THURSDAY	FRIDAY	SATURDAY	SUNDAY
CARDIO							
WEIGHTS							

Weight at beginning of week: Weight at end of week:

Goals for the week:

Ideas for caring, connecting, committing:

HARRY SAYS: DO IT LIKE LANCE ARMSTRONG

I can't emphasize enough the virtues of long, slow training done at 60–65% of max. It may feel so ridiculously easy that you'll wonder what the point is of even getting on the bike. So just remember this: Lance Armstrong did it religiously. I promise you that a 90-minute ride at 60–65% of max is a real part of getting in shape.

Monday␣␣␣␣␣␣␣

How was your night?

Morning mood: Resting Heart Rate:

EXERCISE

CARDIO

Time and/or distance: Level: Heart Rate Max: Recovery:

STRENGTH: UPPER BODY & BACK		STRENGTH: LEGS & ABS	
1:	Reps:	1:	Reps:
2:	Reps:	2:	Reps:
3:	Reps:	3:	Reps:
4:	Reps:	4:	Reps:
5:	Reps:	5:	Reps:

FOOD

Breakfast:

Lunch:

Dinner:

Snacks: Crap: Booze:

LIFE

Caring, connecting, committing:

How did you do? ☐ Amazing ☐ Not Bad ☐ Shameful

Plans for tomorrow:

Tuesday ___ | | |

How was your night?

Morning mood: Resting Heart Rate:

EXERCISE

CARDIO

Time and/or distance: Level: Heart Rate Max: Recovery:

STRENGTH: UPPER BODY & BACK		STRENGTH: LEGS & ABS	
1:	Reps:	1:	Reps:
2:	Reps:	2:	Reps:
3:	Reps:	3:	Reps:
4:	Reps:	4:	Reps:
5:	Reps:	5:	Reps:

FOOD

Breakfast:

Lunch:

Dinner:

Snacks: Crap: Booze:

LIFE

Caring, connecting, committing:

How did you do?   ☐ Amazing   ☐ Not Bad   ☐ Shameful

Plans for tomorrow:

Wednesday ___ | | |

How was your night?

Morning mood: Resting Heart Rate:

EXERCISE

CARDIO

Time and/or distance: Level: Heart Rate Max: Recovery:

STRENGTH: UPPER BODY & BACK		STRENGTH: LEGS & ABS	
1:	Reps:	1:	Reps:
2:	Reps:	2:	Reps:
3:	Reps:	3:	Reps:
4:	Reps:	4:	Reps:
5:	Reps:	5:	Reps:

FOOD

Breakfast:

Lunch:

Dinner:

Snacks: Crap: Booze:

LIFE

Caring, connecting, committing:

How did you do?   ☐ Amazing   ☐ Not Bad   ☐ Shameful

Plans for tomorrow:

Thursday ⌊ | | ⌋

How was your night?

Morning mood: Resting Heart Rate:

EXERCISE

CARDIO

Time and/or distance: Level: Heart Rate Max: Recovery:

STRENGTH: UPPER BODY & BACK		STRENGTH: LEGS & ABS	
1:	Reps:	1:	Reps:
2:	Reps:	2:	Reps:
3:	Reps:	3:	Reps:
4:	Reps:	4:	Reps:
5:	Reps:	5:	Reps:

FOOD

Breakfast:

Lunch:

Dinner:

Snacks: Crap: Booze:

LIFE

Caring, connecting, committing:

How did you do?   ☐ Amazing   ☐ Not Bad   ☐ Shameful

Plans for tomorrow:

Friday ⌊ | | ⌋

How was your night?

Morning mood: Resting Heart Rate:

EXERCISE

CARDIO

Time and/or distance: Level: Heart Rate Max: Recovery:

STRENGTH: UPPER BODY & BACK		STRENGTH: LEGS & ABS	
1:	Reps:	1:	Reps:
2:	Reps:	2:	Reps:
3:	Reps:	3:	Reps:
4:	Reps:	4:	Reps:
5:	Reps:	5:	Reps:

FOOD

Breakfast:

Lunch:

Dinner:

Snacks: Crap: Booze:

LIFE

Caring, connecting, committing:

How did you do?   ☐ Amazing   ☐ Not Bad   ☐ Shameful

Plans for tomorrow:

Saturday ___|___|___

How was your night?

Morning mood: Resting Heart Rate:

CARDIO

Time and/or distance: Level: Heart Rate Max: Recovery:

STRENGTH: UPPER BODY & BACK		STRENGTH: LEGS & ABS	
1:	Reps:	1:	Reps:
2:	Reps:	2:	Reps:
3:	Reps:	3:	Reps:
4:	Reps:	4:	Reps:
5:	Reps:	5:	Reps:

Breakfast:

Lunch:

Dinner:

Snacks: Crap: Booze:

Caring, connecting, committing:

How did you do? ☐ Amazing ☐ Not Bad ☐ Shameful

Plans for tomorrow:

Sunday ___|___|___

How was your night?

Morning mood: Resting Heart Rate:

CARDIO

Time and/or distance: Level: Heart Rate Max: Recovery:

STRENGTH: UPPER BODY & BACK		STRENGTH: LEGS & ABS	
1:	Reps:	1:	Reps:
2:	Reps:	2:	Reps:
3:	Reps:	3:	Reps:
4:	Reps:	4:	Reps:
5:	Reps:	5:	Reps:

Breakfast:

Lunch:

Dinner:

Snacks: Crap: Booze:

Caring, connecting, committing:

How did you do? ☐ Amazing ☐ Not Bad ☐ Shameful

Plans for tomorrow:

Exercise & Diet Plan for the Week

16 week

	MONDAY	TUESDAY	WEDNESDAY	THURSDAY	FRIDAY	SATURDAY	SUNDAY
CARDIO							
WEIGHTS							

Weight at beginning of week: _____ Weight at end of week: _____

Goals for the week:

Ideas for caring, connecting, committing:

CHRIS SAYS: CUSTOMIZE YOUR WORKOUT

Ask your weight trainer to devise a program that will help you get better at one of your favorite sports. Having a goal in mind—whether to be a better skier, tennis player, golfer, you name it—will make it all the more interesting. And believe me, a sports-specific weight-training regimen will help your game (whatever it is) enormously.

Monday

How was your night?

Morning mood: _____ Resting Heart Rate: _____

EXERCISE

CARDIO

Time and/or distance: _____ Level: _____ Heart Rate Max: _____ Recovery: _____

STRENGTH: UPPER BODY & BACK		STRENGTH: LEGS & ABS	
1:	Reps:	1:	Reps:
2:	Reps:	2:	Reps:
3:	Reps:	3:	Reps:
4:	Reps:	4:	Reps:
5:	Reps:	5:	Reps:

FOOD

Breakfast:

Lunch:

Dinner:

Snacks: _____ Crap: _____ Booze: _____

LIFE

Caring, connecting, committing:

How did you do? ☐ Amazing ☐ Not Bad ☐ Shameful

Plans for tomorrow:

Tuesday ___ | | |

How was your night?

Morning mood: Resting Heart Rate:

E X E R C I S E

CARDIO

Time and/or distance: Level: Heart Rate Max: Recovery:

STRENGTH: UPPER BODY & BACK		STRENGTH: LEGS & ABS	
1:	Reps:	1:	Reps:
2:	Reps:	2:	Reps:
3:	Reps:	3:	Reps:
4:	Reps:	4:	Reps:
5:	Reps:	5:	Reps:

F O O D

Breakfast:

Lunch:

Dinner:

Snacks: Crap: Booze:

L I F E

Caring, connecting, committing:

How did you do?   ☐ Amazing   ☐ Not Bad   ☐ Shameful

Plans for tomorrow:

Wednesday ___ | | |

How was your night?

Morning mood: Resting Heart Rate:

E X E R C I S E

CARDIO

Time and/or distance: Level: Heart Rate Max: Recovery:

STRENGTH: UPPER BODY & BACK		STRENGTH: LEGS & ABS	
1:	Reps:	1:	Reps:
2:	Reps:	2:	Reps:
3:	Reps:	3:	Reps:
4:	Reps:	4:	Reps:
5:	Reps:	5:	Reps:

F O O D

Breakfast:

Lunch:

Dinner:

Snacks: Crap: Booze:

L I F E

Caring, connecting, committing:

How did you do?   ☐ Amazing   ☐ Not Bad   ☐ Shameful

Plans for tomorrow:

Thursday ___ | ___ | ___

How was your night?

Morning mood: Resting Heart Rate:

E X E R C I S E

CARDIO

Time and/or distance: Level: Heart Rate Max: Recovery:

STRENGTH: UPPER BODY & BACK		**STRENGTH: LEGS & ABS**	
1:	Reps:	1:	Reps:
2:	Reps:	2:	Reps:
3:	Reps:	3:	Reps:
4:	Reps:	4:	Reps:
5:	Reps:	5:	Reps:

F O O D

Breakfast:

Lunch:

Dinner:

Snacks: Crap: Booze:

L I F E

Caring, connecting, committing:

How did you do?   ☐ Amazing   ☐ Not Bad   ☐ Shameful

Plans for tomorrow:

Friday ___ | ___ | ___

How was your night?

Morning mood: Resting Heart Rate:

E X E R C I S E

CARDIO

Time and/or distance: Level: Heart Rate Max: Recovery:

STRENGTH: UPPER BODY & BACK		**STRENGTH: LEGS & ABS**	
1:	Reps:	1:	Reps:
2:	Reps:	2:	Reps:
3:	Reps:	3:	Reps:
4:	Reps:	4:	Reps:
5:	Reps:	5:	Reps:

F O O D

Breakfast:

Lunch:

Dinner:

Snacks: Crap: Booze:

L I F E

Caring, connecting, committing:

How did you do?   ☐ Amazing   ☐ Not Bad   ☐ Shameful

Plans for tomorrow:

Saturday ___ | | |

How was your night?

Morning mood: ___ Resting Heart Rate:

EXERCISE

CARDIO

Time and/or distance: ___ Level: ___ Heart Rate Max: ___ Recovery:

STRENGTH: UPPER BODY & BACK		STRENGTH: LEGS & ABS	
1:	Reps:	1:	Reps:
2:	Reps:	2:	Reps:
3:	Reps:	3:	Reps:
4:	Reps:	4:	Reps:
5:	Reps:	5:	Reps:

FOOD

Breakfast:

Lunch:

Dinner:

Snacks: ___ Crap: ___ Booze:

LIFE

Caring, connecting, committing:

How did you do? ☐ Amazing ☐ Not Bad ☐ Shameful

Plans for tomorrow.

Sunday ___ | | |

How was your night?

Morning mood: ___ Resting Heart Rate:

EXERCISE

CARDIO

Time and/or distance: ___ Level: ___ Heart Rate Max: ___ Recovery:

STRENGTH: UPPER BODY & BACK		STRENGTH: LEGS & ABS	
1:	Reps:	1:	Reps:
2:	Reps:	2:	Reps:
3:	Reps:	3:	Reps:
4:	Reps:	4:	Reps:
5:	Reps:	5:	Reps:

FOOD

Breakfast:

Lunch:

Dinner:

Snacks: ___ Crap: ___ Booze:

LIFE

Caring, connecting, committing:

How did you do? ☐ Amazing ☐ Not Bad ☐ Shameful

Plans for tomorrow:

Exercise & Diet Plan for the Week

	MONDAY	TUESDAY	WEDNESDAY	THURSDAY	FRIDAY	SATURDAY	SUNDAY
CARDIO							
WEIGHTS							

Weight at beginning of week: _____ Weight at end of week: _____

Goals for the week: _____

Ideas for caring, connecting, committing: _____
_____
_____

HARRY SAYS: **CUT THE CRAP**

Did you know that a McDonald's chicken nuggets and fries combo sold in New York has about ten grams of trans fat (the really bad-for-you stuff), but only one-third of a gram in Denmark? The food industry claims that consumers prefer the taste of trans fat, but I contest that nobody can tell the difference. The real issue is one of economics. But one scientist has estimated that using the healthier fats would increase the cost per order of fries by about a penny. I would happily spend more money to go back to eating fries without guilt, but until that day, I'm going to be careful. You should be, too.

Monday ____ | | |

How was your night? _____

Morning mood: _____ Resting Heart Rate: _____

EXERCISE

CARDIO

Time and/or distance: _____ Level: _____ Heart Rate Max: _____ Recovery: _____

STRENGTH: UPPER BODY & BACK		**STRENGTH: LEGS & ABS**	
1:	Reps:	1:	Reps:
2:	Reps:	2:	Reps:
3:	Reps:	3:	Reps:
4:	Reps:	4:	Reps:
5:	Reps:	5:	Reps:

FOOD

Breakfast:

Lunch:

Dinner:

Snacks: _____ Crap: _____ Booze: _____

LIFE

Caring, connecting, committing:

How did you do? ☐ Amazing ☐ Not Bad ☐ Shameful

Plans for tomorrow:

Tuesday ___ | | |

How was your night?

Morning mood: Resting Heart Rate:

EXERCISE

CARDIO

Time and/or distance: Level: Heart Rate Max: Recovery:

STRENGTH: UPPER BODY & BACK		STRENGTH: LEGS & ABS	
1:	Reps:	1:	Reps:
2:	Reps:	2:	Reps:
3:	Reps:	3:	Reps:
4:	Reps:	4:	Reps:
5:	Reps:	5:	Reps:

FOOD

Breakfast:

Lunch:

Dinner:

Snacks: Crap: Booze:

LIFE

Caring, connecting, committing:

How did you do?   ☐ Amazing   ☐ Not Bad   ☐ Shameful

Plans for tomorrow:

Wednesday ___ | | |

How was your night?

Morning mood: Resting Heart Rate:

EXERCISE

CARDIO

Time and/or distance: Level: Heart Rate Max: Recovery:

STRENGTH: UPPER BODY & BACK		STRENGTH: LEGS & ABS	
1:	Reps:	1:	Reps:
2:	Reps:	2:	Reps:
3:	Reps:	3:	Reps:
4:	Reps:	4:	Reps:
5:	Reps:	5:	Reps:

FOOD

Breakfast:

Lunch:

Dinner:

Snacks: Crap: Booze:

LIFE

Caring, connecting, committing:

How did you do?   ☐ Amazing   ☐ Not Bad   ☐ Shameful

Plans for tomorrow:

Thursday ⎵ | |

How was your night?

Morning mood: Resting Heart Rate:

E X E R C I S E

CARDIO

Time and/or distance: Level: Heart Rate Max: Recovery:

STRENGTH: UPPER BODY & BACK		STRENGTH: LEGS & ABS	
1:	Reps:	1:	Reps:
2:	Reps:	2:	Reps:
3:	Reps:	3:	Reps:
4:	Reps:	4:	Reps:
5:	Reps:	5:	Reps:

F O O D

Breakfast:

Lunch:

Dinner:

Snacks: Crap: Booze:

L I F E

Caring, connecting, committing:

How did you do?   ☐ Amazing   ☐ Not Bad   ☐ Shameful

Plans for tomorrow:

Friday ⎵ | |

How was your night?

Morning mood: Resting Heart Rate:

E X E R C I S E

CARDIO

Time and/or distance: Level: Heart Rate Max: Recovery:

STRENGTH: UPPER BODY & BACK		STRENGTH: LEGS & ABS	
1:	Reps:	1:	Reps:
2:	Reps:	2:	Reps:
3:	Reps:	3:	Reps:
4:	Reps:	4:	Reps:
5:	Reps:	5:	Reps:

F O O D

Breakfast:

Lunch:

Dinner:

Snacks: Crap: Booze:

L I F E

Caring, connecting, committing:

How did you do?   ☐ Amazing   ☐ Not Bad   ☐ Shameful

Plans for tomorrow:

Saturday___|___|___|

How was your night?

Morning mood: Resting Heart Rate:

EXERCISE

CARDIO

Time and/or distance: Level: Heart Rate Max: Recovery:

STRENGTH: UPPER BODY & BACK		STRENGTH: LEGS & ABS	
1:	Reps:	1:	Reps:
2:	Reps:	2:	Reps:
3:	Reps:	3:	Reps:
4:	Reps:	4:	Reps:
5:	Reps:	5:	Reps:

FOOD

Breakfast:

Lunch:

Dinner:

Snacks: Crap: Booze:

LIFE

Caring, connecting, committing:

How did you do?   ☐ Amazing   ☐ Not Bad   ☐ Shameful

Plans for tomorrow:

Sunday___|___|___|

How was your night?

Morning mood: Resting Heart Rate:

EXERCISE

CARDIO

Time and/or distance: Level: Heart Rate Max: Recovery:

STRENGTH: UPPER BODY & BACK		STRENGTH: LEGS & ABS	
1:	Reps:	1:	Reps:
2:	Reps:	2:	Reps:
3:	Reps:	3:	Reps:
4:	Reps:	4:	Reps:
5:	Reps:	5:	Reps:

FOOD

Breakfast:

Lunch:

Dinner:

Snacks: Crap: Booze:

LIFE

Caring, connecting, committing:

How did you do?   ☐ Amazing   ☐ Not Bad   ☐ Shameful

Plans for tomorrow:

Exercise & Diet Plan for the Week

18 week

	MONDAY	TUESDAY	WEDNESDAY	THURSDAY	FRIDAY	SATURDAY	SUNDAY
CARDIO							
WEIGHTS							

Weight at beginning of week: _____ Weight at end of week: _____

Goals for the week:

Ideas for caring, connecting, committing:

CHRIS SAYS: TAP INTO A PASSION

If you're lucky enough to like some athletic activity, make that the basis of your workout regimen. If it's an aerobic sport such as biking or running, all the better—you can do the thing you love for your workouts much of the time. Or train for it . . . spinning class is perfect for those who love to bike. Passion makes the medicine go down. But don't forget to cross train. It's possible to get into a rut. And you can hurt yourself that way.

Monday ___ ___

How was your night? _____

Morning mood: _____ Resting Heart Rate: _____

EXERCISE

CARDIO

Time and/or distance: _____ Level: _____ Heart Rate Max: _____ Recovery: _____

STRENGTH: UPPER BODY & BACK		STRENGTH: LEGS & ABS	
1:	Reps:	1:	Reps:
2:	Reps:	2:	Reps:
3:	Reps:	3:	Reps:
4:	Reps:	4:	Reps:
5:	Reps:	5:	Reps:

FOOD

Breakfast:

Lunch:

Dinner:

Snacks: _____ Crap: _____ Booze: _____

LIFE

Caring, connecting, committing:

How did you do? ☐ Amazing ☐ Not Bad ☐ Shameful

Plans for tomorrow:

Tuesday ___ | | |

How was your night?

Morning mood: Resting Heart Rate:

EXERCISE

CARDIO

Time and/or distance: Level: Heart Rate Max: Recovery:

STRENGTH: UPPER BODY & BACK		STRENGTH: LEGS & ABS	
1:	Reps:	1:	Reps:
2:	Reps:	2:	Reps:
3:	Reps:	3:	Reps:
4:	Reps:	4:	Reps:
5:	Reps:	5:	Reps:

FOOD

Breakfast:

Lunch:

Dinner:

Snacks: Crap: Booze:

LIFE

Caring, connecting, committing:

How did you do?   ☐ Amazing   ☐ Not Bad   ☐ Shameful

Plans for tomorrow:

Wednesday ___ | | |

How was your night?

Morning mood: Resting Heart Rate:

EXERCISE

CARDIO

Time and/or distance: Level: Heart Rate Max: Recovery:

STRENGTH: UPPER BODY & BACK		STRENGTH: LEGS & ABS	
1:	Reps:	1:	Reps:
2:	Reps:	2:	Reps:
3:	Reps:	3:	Reps:
4:	Reps:	4:	Reps:
5:	Reps:	5:	Reps:

FOOD

Breakfast:

Lunch:

Dinner:

Snacks: Crap: Booze:

LIFE

Caring, connecting, committing:

How did you do?   ☐ Amazing   ☐ Not Bad   ☐ Shameful

Plans for tomorrow:

Thursday ⎵ ⎵ ⎵

How was your night?

Morning mood: Resting Heart Rate:

EXERCISE

CARDIO

Time and/or distance: Level: Heart Rate Max: Recovery:

STRENGTH: UPPER BODY & BACK		STRENGTH: LEGS & ABS	
1:	Reps:	1:	Reps:
2:	Reps:	2:	Reps:
3:	Reps:	3:	Reps:
4:	Reps:	4:	Reps:
5:	Reps:	5:	Reps:

FOOD

Breakfast:

Lunch:

Dinner:

Snacks: Crap: Booze:

LIFE

Caring, connecting, committing:

How did you do?   ☐ Amazing   ☐ Not Bad   ☐ Shameful

Plans for tomorrow:

Friday ⎵ ⎵ ⎵

How was your night?

Morning mood: Resting Heart Rate:

EXERCISE

CARDIO

Time and/or distance: Level: Heart Rate Max: Recovery:

STRENGTH: UPPER BODY & BACK		STRENGTH: LEGS & ABS	
1:	Reps:	1:	Reps:
2:	Reps:	2:	Reps:
3:	Reps:	3:	Reps:
4:	Reps:	4:	Reps:
5:	Reps:	5:	Reps:

FOOD

Breakfast:

Lunch:

Dinner:

Snacks: Crap: Booze:

LIFE

Caring, connecting, committing:

How did you do?   ☐ Amazing   ☐ Not Bad   ☐ Shameful

Plans for tomorrow:

Saturday ___|___|___

How was your night?

Morning mood: Resting Heart Rate:

E X E R C I S E

CARDIO

Time and/or distance: Level: Heart Rate Max: Recovery:

STRENGTH: UPPER BODY & BACK	STRENGTH: LEGS & ABS
1: Reps:	1: Reps:
2: Reps:	2: Reps:
3: Reps:	3: Reps:
4: Reps:	4: Reps:
5: Reps:	5: Reps:

F O O D

Breakfast:

Lunch:

Dinner:

Snacks: Crap: Booze:

L I F E

Caring, connecting, committing:

How did you do?   ☐ Amazing ☐ Not Bad ☐ Shameful

Plans for tomorrow:

Sunday ___|___|___

How was your night?

Morning mood: Resting Heart Rate:

E X E R C I S E

CARDIO

Time and/or distance: Level: Heart Rate Max: Recovery:

STRENGTH: UPPER BODY & BACK	STRENGTH: LEGS & ABS
1: Reps:	1: Reps:
2: Reps:	2: Reps:
3: Reps:	3: Reps:
4: Reps:	4: Reps:
5: Reps:	5: Reps:

F O O D

Breakfast:

Lunch:

Dinner:

Snacks: Crap: Booze:

L I F E

Caring, connecting, committing:

How did you do?   ☐ Amazing ☐ Not Bad ☐ Shameful

Plans for tomorrow:

19 week

Exercise & Diet Plan for the Week

	MONDAY	TUESDAY	WEDNESDAY	THURSDAY	FRIDAY	SATURDAY	SUNDAY
CARDIO							
WEIGHTS							

Weight at beginning of week: _____ Weight at end of week: _____

Goals for the week:

Ideas for caring, connecting, committing:

HARRY SAYS: **HEAD FOR THE HILLS**

There are wonderful hidden walks everywhere, but if you have a choice, look for some hills to climb. The challenge and variety will do you good. We all should be covering the equivalent of three to six miles a day—which is farther than you think. If you're in doubt, get a pedometer. Then have some fun. And don't forget to daydream.

Monday ☐ ☐ ☐

How was your night?

Morning mood: _____ Resting Heart Rate: _____

EXERCISE

CARDIO

Time and/or distance: _____ Level: _____ Heart Rate Max: _____ Recovery: _____

STRENGTH: UPPER BODY & BACK		STRENGTH: LEGS & ABS	
1:	Reps:	1:	Reps:
2:	Reps:	2:	Reps:
3:	Reps:	3:	Reps:
4:	Reps:	4:	Reps:
5:	Reps:	5:	Reps:

FOOD

Breakfast:

Lunch:

Dinner:

Snacks: _____ Crap: _____ Booze: _____

LIFE

Caring, connecting, committing:

How did you do? ☐ Amazing ☐ Not Bad ☐ Shameful

Plans for tomorrow:

Tuesday_____

How was your night?

Morning mood: Resting Heart Rate:

EXERCISE

CARDIO

Time and/or distance: Level: Heart Rate Max: Recovery:

STRENGTH: UPPER BODY & BACK		**STRENGTH: LEGS & ABS**	
1:	Reps:	1:	Reps:
2:	Reps:	2:	Reps:
3:	Reps:	3:	Reps:
4:	Reps:	4:	Reps:
5:	Reps:	5:	Reps:

FOOD

Breakfast:

Lunch:

Dinner:

Snacks: Crap: Booze:

LIFE

Caring, connecting, committing:

How did you do?   ☐ Amazing   ☐ Not Bad   ☐ Shameful

Plans for tomorrow:

Wednesday_____

How was your night?

Morning mood: Resting Heart Rate:

EXERCISE

CARDIO

Time and/or distance: Level: Heart Rate Max: Recovery:

STRENGTH: UPPER BODY & BACK		**STRENGTH: LEGS & ABS**	
1:	Reps:	1:	Reps:
2:	Reps:	2:	Reps:
3:	Reps:	3:	Reps:
4:	Reps:	4:	Reps:
5:	Reps:	5:	Reps:

FOOD

Breakfast:

Lunch:

Dinner:

Snacks: Crap: Booze:

LIFE

Caring, connecting, committing:

How did you do?   ☐ Amazing   ☐ Not Bad   ☐ Shameful

Plans for tomorrow:

Thursday _ | | |

How was your night?

Morning mood: Resting Heart Rate:

E X E R C I S E

CARDIO

Time and/or distance: Level: Heart Rate Max: Recovery:

STRENGTH: UPPER BODY & BACK		**STRENGTH: LEGS & ABS**	
1:	Reps:	1:	Reps:
2:	Reps:	2:	Reps:
3:	Reps:	3:	Reps:
4:	Reps:	4:	Reps:
5:	Reps:	5:	Reps:

F O O D

Breakfast:

Lunch:

Dinner:

Snacks: Crap: Booze:

L I F E

Caring, connecting, committing:

How did you do?   ☐ Amazing ☐ Not Bad ☐ Shameful

Plans for tomorrow:

Friday _ | | |

How was your night?

Morning mood: Resting Heart Rate:

E X E R C I S E

CARDIO

Time and/or distance: Level: Heart Rate Max: Recovery:

STRENGTH: UPPER BODY & BACK		**STRENGTH: LEGS & ABS**	
1:	Reps:	1:	Reps:
2:	Reps:	2:	Reps:
3:	Reps:	3:	Reps:
4:	Reps:	4:	Reps:
5:	Reps:	5:	Reps:

F O O D

Breakfast:

Lunch:

Dinner:

Snacks: Crap: Booze:

L I F E

Caring, connecting, committing:

How did you do?   ☐ Amazing ☐ Not Bad ☐ Shameful

Plans for tomorrow:

Saturday___|__|__|

How was your night?

Morning mood: Resting Heart Rate:

EXERCISE

CARDIO

Time and/or distance: Level: Heart Rate Max: Recovery:

STRENGTH: UPPER BODY & BACK		STRENGTH: LEGS & ABS	
1:	Reps:	1:	Reps:
2:	Reps:	2:	Reps:
3:	Reps:	3:	Reps:
4:	Reps:	4:	Reps:
5:	Reps:	5:	Reps:

FOOD

Breakfast:

Lunch:

Dinner:

Snacks: Crap: Booze:

LIFE

Caring, connecting, committing:

How did you do?   ☐ Amazing   ☐ Not Bad   ☐ Shameful

Plans for tomorrow:

Sunday___|__|__|

How was your night?

Morning mood: Resting Heart Rate:

EXERCISE

CARDIO

Time and/or distance: Level: Heart Rate Max: Recovery:

STRENGTH: UPPER BODY & BACK		STRENGTH: LEGS & ABS	
1:	Reps:	1:	Reps:
2:	Reps:	2:	Reps:
3:	Reps:	3:	Reps:
4:	Reps:	4:	Reps:
5:	Reps:	5:	Reps:

FOOD

Breakfast:

Lunch:

Dinner:

Snacks: Crap: Booze:

LIFE

Caring, connecting, committing:

How did you do?   ☐ Amazing   ☐ Not Bad   ☐ Shameful

Plans for tomorrow:

20
week

Exercise & Diet Plan for the Week

	MONDAY	TUESDAY	WEDNESDAY	THURSDAY	FRIDAY	SATURDAY	SUNDAY
CARDIO							
WEIGHTS							

Weight at beginning of week: _____ Weight at end of week: _____

Goals for the week: _____

Ideas for caring, connecting, committing: _____

CHRIS SAYS: GO FOR IT!

Okay, quit daydreaming. You've been doing this stuff for a while now, right? Your aerobic base is not bad . . . you can go at 65% to 75% of your max for an hour and a half, yes? Your doctor says it's okay to go really hard? Start doing intervals. Go at an all-out sprint for thirty seconds, say 95% of your max. Rest a minute. Do it again. Once you have been doing this for a few weeks, try going at 100% of your peak effort for the last ten seconds and you will find your true maximum heart rate. Try this once a week or so. It feels good. If you like it, go to the website to learn more.

Monday ___ | | |

How was your night? _____

Morning mood: _____ Resting Heart Rate: _____

E X E R C I S E

CARDIO

Time and/or distance: _____ Level: _____ Heart Rate Max: _____ Recovery: _____

STRENGTH: UPPER BODY & BACK		STRENGTH: LEGS & ABS	
1:	Reps:	1:	Reps:
2:	Reps:	2:	Reps:
3:	Reps:	3:	Reps:
4:	Reps:	4:	Reps:
5:	Reps:	5:	Reps:

F O O D

Breakfast:

Lunch:

Dinner:

Snacks: _____ Crap: _____ Booze: _____

L I F E

Caring, connecting, committing:

How did you do? ☐ Amazing ☐ Not Bad ☐ Shameful

Plans for tomorrow:

Tuesday___|__|__|

How was your night?

Morning mood: Resting Heart Rate:

EXERCISE

CARDIO

Time and/or distance: Level: Heart Rate Max: Recovery:

STRENGTH: UPPER BODY & BACK		STRENGTH: LEGS & ABS	
1:	Reps:	1:	Reps:
2:	Reps:	2:	Reps:
3:	Reps:	3:	Reps:
4:	Reps:	4:	Reps:
5:	Reps:	5:	Reps:

FOOD

Breakfast:

Lunch:

Dinner:

Snacks: Crap: Booze:

LIFE

Caring, connecting, committing:

How did you do? ☐ Amazing ☐ Not Bad ☐ Shameful

Plans for tomorrow:

Wednesday___|__|__|

How was your night?

Morning mood: Resting Heart Rate:

EXERCISE

CARDIO

Time and/or distance: Level: Heart Rate Max: Recovery:

STRENGTH: UPPER BODY & BACK		STRENGTH: LEGS & ABS	
1:	Reps:	1:	Reps:
2:	Reps:	2:	Reps:
3:	Reps:	3:	Reps:
4:	Reps:	4:	Reps:
5:	Reps:	5:	Reps:

FOOD

Breakfast:

Lunch:

Dinner:

Snacks: Crap: Booze:

LIFE

Caring, connecting, committing:

How did you do? ☐ Amazing ☐ Not Bad ☐ Shameful

Plans for tomorrow:

Thursday ___ | | |

How was your night?

Morning mood: Resting Heart Rate:

E X E R C I S E

CARDIO

Time and/or distance: Level: Heart Rate Max: Recovery:

STRENGTH: UPPER BODY & BACK		**STRENGTH: LEGS & ABS**	
1:	Reps:	1:	Reps:
2:	Reps:	2:	Reps:
3:	Reps:	3:	Reps:
4:	Reps:	4:	Reps:
5:	Reps:	5:	Reps:

F O O D

Breakfast:

Lunch:

Dinner:

Snacks: Crap: Booze:

L I F E

Caring, connecting, committing:

How did you do?   ☐ Amazing   ☐ Not Bad   ☐ Shameful

Plans for tomorrow:

Friday ___ | | |

How was your night?

Morning mood: Resting Heart Rate:

E X E R C I S E

CARDIO

Time and/or distance: Level: Heart Rate Max: Recovery:

STRENGTH: UPPER BODY & BACK		**STRENGTH: LEGS & ABS**	
1:	Reps:	1:	Reps:
2:	Reps:	2:	Reps:
3:	Reps:	3:	Reps:
4:	Reps:	4:	Reps:
5:	Reps:	5:	Reps:

F O O D

Breakfast:

Lunch:

Dinner:

Snacks: Crap: Booze:

L I F E

Caring, connecting, committing:

How did you do?   ☐ Amazing   ☐ Not Bad   ☐ Shameful

Plans for tomorrow:

Saturday_ | | |

How was your night?

Morning mood: | Resting Heart Rate:

EXERCISE

CARDIO

Time and/or distance: | Level: | Heart Rate Max: | Recovery:

STRENGTH: UPPER BODY & BACK		STRENGTH: LEGS & ABS	
1:	Reps:	1:	Reps:
2:	Reps:	2:	Reps:
3:	Reps:	3:	Reps:
4:	Reps:	4:	Reps:
5:	Reps:	5:	Reps:

FOOD

Breakfast:

Lunch:

Dinner:

Snacks: | Crap: | Booze:

LIFE

Caring, connecting, committing:

How did you do? ☐ Amazing ☐ Not Bad ☐ Shameful

Plans for tomorrow:

Sunday_ | | |

How was your night?

Morning mood: | Resting Heart Rate:

EXERCISE

CARDIO

Time and/or distance: | Level: | Heart Rate Max: | Recovery:

STRENGTH: UPPER BODY & BACK		STRENGTH: LEGS & ABS	
1:	Reps:	1:	Reps:
2:	Reps:	2:	Reps:
3:	Reps:	3:	Reps:
4:	Reps:	4:	Reps:
5:	Reps:	5:	Reps:

FOOD

Breakfast:

Lunch:

Dinner:

Snacks: | Crap: | Booze:

LIFE

Caring, connecting, committing:

How did you do? ☐ Amazing ☐ Not Bad ☐ Shameful

Plans for tomorrow:

Exercise & Diet Plan for the Week

	MONDAY	TUESDAY	WEDNESDAY	THURSDAY	FRIDAY	SATURDAY	SUNDAY
CARDIO							
WEIGHTS							

Weight at beginning of week: Weight at end of week:

Goals for the week:

Ideas for caring, connecting, committing:

HARRY SAYS: TAKE IT EASY IF YOU NEED TO

If your heart rate is close to 70% of your theoretical max even when you're doing very little, you are probably really out of shape. If that's the case, go for "long and slow" (at 60% of your max) for six weeks or so. Once you get into somewhat better shape, you can begin pushing yourself harder. But since there may be something going on in your body that is bringing up your heart rate, you should absolutely check with your physician before carrying on the exercise program. If you get the green light, just be prepared to go excruciatingly slow for a while. Trust me: You will improve.

Monday ___ | | |

How was your night?

Morning mood: Resting Heart Rate:

E X E R C I S E

CARDIO

Time and/or distance: Level: Heart Rate Max: Recovery:

STRENGTH: UPPER BODY & BACK		STRENGTH: LEGS & ABS	
1:	Reps:	1:	Reps:
2:	Reps:	2:	Reps:
3:	Reps:	3:	Reps:
4:	Reps:	4:	Reps:
5:	Reps:	5:	Reps:

F O O D

Breakfast:

Lunch:

Dinner:

Snacks: Crap: Booze:

L I F E

Caring, connecting, committing:

How did you do? ☐ Amazing ☐ Not Bad ☐ Shameful

Plans for tomorrow:

Tuesday ___ | | |

How was your night?

Morning mood: Resting Heart Rate:

E X E R C I S E

CARDIO

Time and/or distance: Level: Heart Rate Max: Recovery:

STRENGTH: UPPER BODY & BACK		STRENGTH: LEGS & ABS	
1:	Reps:	1:	Reps:
2:	Reps:	2:	Reps:
3:	Reps:	3:	Reps:
4:	Reps:	4:	Reps:
5:	Reps:	5:	Reps:

F O O D

Breakfast:

Lunch:

Dinner:

Snacks: Crap: Booze:

L I F E

Caring, connecting, committing:

How did you do?   ☐ Amazing   ☐ Not Bad   ☐ Shameful

Plans for tomorrow:

Wednesday ___ | | |

How was your night?

Morning mood: Resting Heart Rate:

E X E R C I S E

CARDIO

Time and/or distance: Level: Heart Rate Max: Recovery:

STRENGTH: UPPER BODY & BACK		STRENGTH: LEGS & ABS	
1:	Reps:	1:	Reps:
2:	Reps:	2:	Reps:
3:	Reps:	3:	Reps:
4:	Reps:	4:	Reps:
5:	Reps:	5:	Reps:

F O O D

Breakfast:

Lunch:

Dinner:

Snacks: Crap: Booze:

L I F E

Caring, connecting, committing:

How did you do?   ☐ Amazing   ☐ Not Bad   ☐ Shameful

Plans for tomorrow:

Thursday ___ | | |

How was your night?

Morning mood: Resting Heart Rate:

EXERCISE

CARDIO

Time and/or distance: Level: Heart Rate Max: Recovery:

STRENGTH: UPPER BODY & BACK		STRENGTH: LEGS & ABS	
1:	Reps:	1:	Reps:
2:	Reps:	2:	Reps:
3:	Reps:	3:	Reps:
4:	Reps:	4:	Reps:
5:	Reps:	5:	Reps:

FOOD

Breakfast:

Lunch:

Dinner:

Snacks: Crap: Booze:

LIFE

Caring, connecting, committing:

How did you do?   ☐ Amazing ☐ Not Bad ☐ Shameful

Plans for tomorrow:

Friday ___ | | |

How was your night?

Morning mood: Resting Heart Rate:

EXERCISE

CARDIO

Time and/or distance: Level: Heart Rate Max: Recovery:

STRENGTH: UPPER BODY & BACK		STRENGTH: LEGS & ABS	
1:	Reps:	1:	Reps:
2:	Reps:	2:	Reps:
3:	Reps:	3:	Reps:
4:	Reps:	4:	Reps:
5:	Reps:	5:	Reps:

FOOD

Breakfast:

Lunch:

Dinner:

Snacks: Crap: Booze:

LIFE

Caring, connecting, committing:

How did you do?   ☐ Amazing ☐ Not Bad ☐ Shameful

Plans for tomorrow:

Saturday _ _ _

How was your night?

Morning mood: Resting Heart Rate:

E X E R C I S E

CARDIO

Time and/or distance: Level: Heart Rate Max: Recovery:

STRENGTH: UPPER BODY & BACK		STRENGTH: LEGS & ABS	
1:	Reps:	1:	Reps:
2:	Reps:	2:	Reps:
3:	Reps:	3:	Reps:
4:	Reps:	4:	Reps:
5:	Reps:	5:	Reps:

F O O D

Breakfast:

Lunch:

Dinner:

Snacks: Crap: Booze:

L I F E

Caring, connecting, committing:

How did you do? ☐ Amazing ☐ Not Bad ☐ Shameful

Plans for tomorrow:

Sunday _ _ _

How was your night?

Morning mood: Resting Heart Rate:

E X E R C I S E

CARDIO

Time and/or distance: Level: Heart Rate Max: Recovery:

STRENGTH: UPPER BODY & BACK		STRENGTH: LEGS & ABS	
1:	Reps:	1:	Reps:
2:	Reps:	2:	Reps:
3:	Reps:	3:	Reps:
4:	Reps:	4:	Reps:
5:	Reps:	5:	Reps:

F O O D

Breakfast:

Lunch:

Dinner:

Snacks: Crap: Booze:

L I F E

Caring, connecting, committing:

How did you do? ☐ Amazing ☐ Not Bad ☐ Shameful

Plans for tomorrow:

22 week | Exercise & Diet Plan for the Week

	MONDAY	TUESDAY	WEDNESDAY	THURSDAY	FRIDAY	SATURDAY	SUNDAY
CARDIO							
WEIGHTS							

Weight at beginning of week: _____ Weight at end of week: _____

Goals for the week:

Ideas for caring, connecting, committing:

CHRIS SAYS: NEVER QUIT

There'll be days when you hate and dread the idea of going to the gym. Well, suck it up and go anyway. And if you fall apart completely and do not go today or this week, go the next day! And the day after that! NEVER QUIT. EVER.

Monday ___ ___

How was your night?

Morning mood: _____ Resting Heart Rate: _____

EXERCISE

CARDIO

Time and/or distance: _____ Level: _____ Heart Rate Max: _____ Recovery: _____

STRENGTH: UPPER BODY & BACK		STRENGTH: LEGS & ABS	
1:	Reps:	1:	Reps:
2:	Reps:	2:	Reps:
3:	Reps:	3:	Reps:
4:	Reps:	4:	Reps:
5:	Reps:	5:	Reps:

FOOD

Breakfast:

Lunch:

Dinner:

Snacks: _____ Crap: _____ Booze: _____

LIFE

Caring, connecting, committing:

How did you do? ☐ Amazing ☐ Not Bad ☐ Shameful

Plans for tomorrow:

Tuesday __ | | |

How was your night?	
Morning mood:	Resting Heart Rate:

EXERCISE

CARDIO

Time and/or distance: Level: Heart Rate Max: Recovery:

STRENGTH: UPPER BODY & BACK		STRENGTH: LEGS & ABS	
1:	Reps:	1:	Reps:
2:	Reps:	2:	Reps:
3:	Reps:	3:	Reps:
4:	Reps:	4:	Reps:
5:	Reps:	5:	Reps:

FOOD

Breakfast:

Lunch:

Dinner:

Snacks: Crap: Booze:

LIFE

Caring, connecting, committing:

How did you do? ☐ Amazing ☐ Not Bad ☐ Shameful

Plans for tomorrow:

Wednesday __ | |

How was your night?	
Morning mood:	Resting Heart Rate:

EXERCISE

CARDIO

Time and/or distance: Level: Heart Rate Max: Recovery:

STRENGTH: UPPER BODY & BACK		STRENGTH: LEGS & ABS	
1:	Reps:	1:	Reps:
2:	Reps:	2:	Reps:
3:	Reps:	3:	Reps:
4:	Reps:	4:	Reps:
5:	Reps:	5:	Reps:

FOOD

Breakfast:

Lunch:

Dinner:

Snacks: Crap: Booze:

LIFE

Caring, connecting, committing:

How did you do? ☐ Amazing ☐ Not Bad ☐ Shameful

Plans for tomorrow:

Thursday ⊔⊔⊔

How was your night?

Morning mood: Resting Heart Rate:

EXERCISE

CARDIO

Time and/or distance: Level: Heart Rate Max: Recovery:

STRENGTH: UPPER BODY & BACK		STRENGTH: LEGS & ABS	
1:	Reps:	1:	Reps:
2:	Reps:	2:	Reps:
3:	Reps:	3:	Reps:
4:	Reps:	4:	Reps:
5:	Reps:	5:	Reps:

FOOD

Breakfast:

Lunch:

Dinner:

Snacks: Crap: Booze:

LIFE

Caring, connecting, committing:

How did you do? ☐ Amazing ☐ Not Bad ☐ Shameful

Plans for tomorrow:

Friday ⊔⊔⊔

How was your night?

Morning mood: Resting Heart Rate:

EXERCISE

CARDIO

Time and/or distance: Level: Heart Rate Max: Recovery:

STRENGTH: UPPER BODY & BACK		STRENGTH: LEGS & ABS	
1:	Reps:	1:	Reps:
2:	Reps:	2:	Reps:
3:	Reps:	3:	Reps:
4:	Reps:	4:	Reps:
5:	Reps:	5:	Reps:

FOOD

Breakfast:

Lunch:

Dinner:

Snacks: Crap: Booze:

LIFE

Caring, connecting, committing:

How did you do? ☐ Amazing ☐ Not Bad ☐ Shameful

Plans for tomorrow:

Saturday ___|___|___

How was your night?

Morning mood: Resting Heart Rate:

EXERCISE

CARDIO

Time and/or distance: Level: Heart Rate Max: Recovery:

STRENGTH: UPPER BODY & BACK		STRENGTH: LEGS & ABS	
1:	Reps:	1:	Reps:
2:	Reps:	2:	Reps:
3:	Reps:	3:	Reps:
4:	Reps:	4:	Reps:
5:	Reps:	5:	Reps:

FOOD

Breakfast:

Lunch:

Dinner:

Snacks: Crap: Booze:

LIFE

Caring, connecting, committing:

How did you do? ☐ Amazing ☐ Not Bad ☐ Shameful

Plans for tomorrow:

Sunday ___|___|___

How was your night?

Morning mood: Resting Heart Rate:

EXERCISE

CARDIO

Time and/or distance: Level: Heart Rate Max: Recovery:

STRENGTH: UPPER BODY & BACK		STRENGTH: LEGS & ABS	
1:	Reps:	1:	Reps:
2:	Reps:	2:	Reps:
3:	Reps:	3:	Reps:
4:	Reps:	4:	Reps:
5:	Reps:	5:	Reps:

FOOD

Breakfast:

Lunch:

Dinner:

Snacks: Crap: Booze:

LIFE

Caring, connecting, committing:

How did you do? ☐ Amazing ☐ Not Bad ☐ Shameful

Plans for tomorrow:

23 week

Exercise & Diet Plan for the Week

	MONDAY	TUESDAY	WEDNESDAY	THURSDAY	FRIDAY	SATURDAY	SUNDAY
CARDIO							
WEIGHTS							

Weight at beginning of week: _____ Weight at end of week: _____

Goals for the week:

Ideas for caring, connecting, committing:

HARRY SAYS: **GET THE MOST OUT OF GOLF**

Chris is skeptical, but there really is a way to make golf count as low-intensity aerobic activity. Walk vigorously for eighteen holes and pull your own clubs. But here's the rub: Most people move at the pace of their slowest golf buddy, turning a game into more of an extended stroll than actual exercise. So have fun, but don't fool yourself.

Monday | | |

How was your night?

Morning mood: _____ Resting Heart Rate: _____

EXERCISE

CARDIO

Time and/or distance: _____ Level: _____ Heart Rate Max: _____ Recovery: _____

STRENGTH: UPPER BODY & BACK		**STRENGTH: LEGS & ABS**	
1:	Reps:	1:	Reps:
2:	Reps:	2:	Reps:
3:	Reps:	3:	Reps:
4:	Reps:	4:	Reps:
5:	Reps:	5:	Reps:

FOOD

Breakfast:

Lunch:

Dinner:

Snacks: _____ Crap: _____ Booze: _____

LIFE

Caring, connecting, committing:

How did you do? ☐ Amazing ☐ Not Bad ☐ Shameful

Plans for tomorrow:

Tuesday ⎵ ⎵ ⎵

How was your night?

Morning mood: Resting Heart Rate:

EXERCISE

CARDIO

Time and/or distance: Level: Heart Rate Max: Recovery:

STRENGTH: UPPER BODY & BACK		STRENGTH: LEGS & ABS	
1:	Reps:	1:	Reps:
2:	Reps:	2:	Reps:
3:	Reps:	3:	Reps:
4:	Reps:	4:	Reps:
5:	Reps:	5:	Reps:

FOOD

Breakfast:

Lunch:

Dinner:

Snacks: Crap: Booze:

LIFE

Caring, connecting, committing:

How did you do? ☐ Amazing ☐ Not Bad ☐ Shameful

Plans for tomorrow:

Wednesday ⎵ ⎵ ⎵

How was your night?

Morning mood: Resting Heart Rate:

EXERCISE

CARDIO

Time and/or distance: Level: Heart Rate Max: Recovery:

STRENGTH: UPPER BODY & BACK		STRENGTH: LEGS & ABS	
1:	Reps:	1:	Reps:
2:	Reps:	2:	Reps:
3:	Reps:	3:	Reps:
4:	Reps:	4:	Reps:
5:	Reps:	5:	Reps:

FOOD

Breakfast:

Lunch:

Dinner:

Snacks: Crap: Booze:

LIFE

Caring, connecting, committing:

How did you do? ☐ Amazing ☐ Not Bad ☐ Shameful

Plans for tomorrow:

Thursday ⌐ | | ⌐

How was your night?

Morning mood: Resting Heart Rate:

E X E R C I S E

CARDIO

Time and/or distance: Level: Heart Rate Max: Recovery:

STRENGTH: UPPER BODY & BACK		STRENGTH: LEGS & ABS	
1:	Reps:	1:	Reps:
2:	Reps:	2:	Reps:
3:	Reps:	3:	Reps:
4:	Reps:	4:	Reps:
5:	Reps:	5:	Reps:

F O O D

Breakfast:

Lunch:

Dinner:

Snacks: Crap: Booze:

L I F E

Caring, connecting, committing:

How did you do?   ☐ Amazing   ☐ Not Bad   ☐ Shameful

Plans for tomorrow:

Friday ⌐ | | ⌐

How was your night?

Morning mood: Resting Heart Rate:

E X E R C I S E

CARDIO

Time and/or distance: Level: Heart Rate Max: Recovery:

STRENGTH: UPPER BODY & BACK		STRENGTH: LEGS & ABS	
1:	Reps:	1:	Reps:
2:	Reps:	2:	Reps:
3:	Reps:	3:	Reps:
4:	Reps:	4:	Reps:
5:	Reps:	5:	Reps:

F O O D

Breakfast:

Lunch:

Dinner:

Snacks: Crap: Booze:

L I F E

Caring, connecting, committing:

How did you do?   ☐ Amazing   ☐ Not Bad   ☐ Shameful

Plans for tomorrow:

Saturday _ | _ | _ |

How was your night?

Morning mood: Resting Heart Rate:

E X E R C I S E

CARDIO

Time and/or distance: Level: Heart Rate Max: Recovery:

STRENGTH: UPPER BODY & BACK		STRENGTH: LEGS & ABS	
1:	Reps:	1:	Reps:
2:	Reps:	2:	Reps:
3:	Reps:	3:	Reps:
4:	Reps:	4:	Reps:
5:	Reps:	5:	Reps:

F O O D

Breakfast:

Lunch:

Dinner:

Snacks: Crap: Booze:

L I F E

Caring, connecting, committing:

How did you do?   ☐ Amazing   ☐ Not Bad   ☐ Shameful

Plans for tomorrow:

Sunday _ | _ | _ |

How was your night?

Morning mood: Resting Heart Rate:

E X E R C I S E

CARDIO

Time and/or distance: Level: Heart Rate Max: Recovery:

STRENGTH: UPPER BODY & BACK		STRENGTH: LEGS & ABS	
1:	Reps:	1:	Reps:
2:	Reps:	2:	Reps:
3:	Reps:	3:	Reps:
4:	Reps:	4:	Reps:
5:	Reps:	5:	Reps:

F O O D

Breakfast:

Lunch:

Dinner:

Snacks: Crap: Booze:

L I F E

Caring, connecting, committing:

How did you do?   ☐ Amazing   ☐ Not Bad   ☐ Shameful

Plans for tomorrow:

Exercise & Diet Plan for the Week

	MONDAY	TUESDAY	WEDNESDAY	THURSDAY	FRIDAY	SATURDAY	SUNDAY
CARDIO							
WEIGHTS							

Weight at beginning of week: Weight at end of week:

Goals for the week:

Ideas for caring, connecting, committing:

CHRIS SAYS: GOLF? PUH-LEASE!

Golf is a hell of a game. Obviously. But aerobic? I don't see it. Maybe if you crawl around the course on your hands and knees. Or put a fifty-pound weight in your bag. But mostly it's fun. And the social contact is worth a lot. But it ain't aerobic. Unless you *fly*. And, let's face it, most of you aren't flying. Check it out by walking the course while you're wearing a heart rate monitor. You'll see.

Monday ___ ___ ___

How was your night?

Morning mood: Resting Heart Rate:

E X E R C I S E

CARDIO

Time and/or distance: Level: Heart Rate Max: Recovery:

STRENGTH: UPPER BODY & BACK		STRENGTH: LEGS & ABS	
1:	Reps:	1:	Reps:
2:	Reps:	2:	Reps:
3:	Reps:	3:	Reps:
4:	Reps:	4:	Reps:
5:	Reps:	5:	Reps:

F O O D

Breakfast:

Lunch:

Dinner:

Snacks: Crap: Booze:

L I F E

Caring, connecting, committing:

How did you do? ☐ Amazing ☐ Not Bad ☐ Shameful

Plans for tomorrow:

Tuesday ___ | | |

How was your night?

Morning mood: Resting Heart Rate:

E X E R C I S E

CARDIO

Time and/or distance: Level: Heart Rate Max: Recovery:

STRENGTH: UPPER BODY & BACK		STRENGTH: LEGS & ABS	
1:	Reps:	1:	Reps:
2:	Reps:	2:	Reps:
3:	Reps:	3:	Reps:
4:	Reps:	4:	Reps:
5:	Reps:	5:	Reps:

F o o n

Breakfast:

Lunch:

Dinner:

Snacks: Crap: Booze:

L I F E

Caring, connecting, committing:

How did you do?   ☐ Amazing ☐ Not Bad ☐ Shameful

Plans for tomorrow:

Wednesday ___ | | |

How was your night?

Morning mood: Resting Heart Rate:

E X E R C I S E

CARDIO

Time and/or distance: Level: Heart Rate Max: Recovery:

STRENGTH: UPPER BODY & BACK		STRENGTH: LEGS & ABS	
1:	Reps:	1:	Reps:
2:	Reps:	2:	Reps:
3:	Reps:	3:	Reps:
4:	Reps:	4:	Reps:
5:	Reps:	5:	Reps:

F o o D

Breakfast:

Lunch:

Dinner:

Snacks: Crap: Booze:

L I F E

Caring, connecting, committing:

How did you do?   ☐ Amazing ☐ Not Bad ☐ Shameful

Plans for tomorrow:

Thursday___|__|___|

How was your night?

Morning mood: Resting Heart Rate:

EXERCISE

CARDIO

Time and/or distance: Level: Heart Rate Max: Recovery:

STRENGTH: UPPER BODY & BACK		STRENGTH: LEGS & ABS	
1:	Reps:	1:	Reps:
2:	Reps:	2:	Reps:
3:	Reps:	3:	Reps:
4:	Reps:	4:	Reps:
5:	Reps:	5:	Reps:

FOOD

Breakfast:

Lunch:

Dinner:

Snacks: Crap: Booze:

LIFE

Caring, connecting, committing:

How did you do?   ☐ Amazing ☐ Not Bad ☐ Shameful

Plans for tomorrow:

Friday___|__|___|

How was your night?

Morning mood: Resting Heart Rate:

EXERCISE

CARDIO

Time and/or distance: Level: Heart Rate Max: Recovery:

STRENGTH: UPPER BODY & BACK		STRENGTH: LEGS & ABS	
1:	Reps:	1:	Reps:
2:	Reps:	2:	Reps:
3:	Reps:	3:	Reps:
4:	Reps:	4:	Reps:
5:	Reps:	5:	Reps:

FOOD

Breakfast:

Lunch:

Dinner:

Snacks: Crap: Booze:

LIFE

Caring, connecting, committing:

How did you do?   ☐ Amazing ☐ Not Bad ☐ Shameful

Plans for tomorrow:

Saturday _ | | |

How was your night?

Morning mood: Resting Heart Rate:

EXERCISE

CARDIO

Time and/or distance: Level: Heart Rate Max: Recovery:

STRENGTH: UPPER BODY & BACK		STRENGTH: LEGS & ABS	
1:	Reps:	1:	Reps:
2:	Reps:	2:	Reps:
3:	Reps:	3:	Reps:
4:	Reps:	4:	Reps:
5:	Reps:	5:	Reps:

FOOD

Breakfast:

Lunch:

Dinner:

Snacks: Crap: Booze:

LIFE

Caring, connecting, committing:

How did you do? ☐ Amazing ☐ Not Bad ☐ Shameful

Plans for tomorrow:

Sunday _ | | |

How was your night?

Morning mood: Resting Heart Rate:

EXERCISE

CARDIO

Time and/or distance: Level: Heart Rate Max: Recovery:

STRENGTH: UPPER BODY & BACK		STRENGTH: LEGS & ABS	
1:	Reps:	1:	Reps:
2:	Reps:	2:	Reps:
3:	Reps:	3:	Reps:
4:	Reps:	4:	Reps:
5:	Reps:	5:	Reps:

FOOD

Breakfast:

Lunch:

Dinner:

Snacks: Crap: Booze:

LIFE

Caring, connecting, committing:

How did you do? ☐ Amazing ☐ Not Bad ☐ Shameful

Plans for tomorrow:

Exercise & Diet Plan for the Week

	MONDAY	TUESDAY	WEDNESDAY	THURSDAY	FRIDAY	SATURDAY	SUNDAY
CARDIO							
WEIGHTS							

Weight at beginning of week: Weight at end of week:

Goals for the week:

Ideas for caring, connecting, committing:

HARRY SAYS: PAY ATTENTION TO YOUR RESTING PULSE

If you're feeling particularly tired, your body may be asking you for a chance to restore itself. Check your resting pulse first thing in the morning, while you're still in bed. If it is up over your baseline, your body needs some more low-intensity training. Try going at an easy pace (60% of your maximum heart rate) two days a week to let your body recover from your more intense workouts.

Monday

How was your night?

Morning mood: Resting Heart Rate:

E X E R C I S E

CARDIO

Time and/or distance: Level: Heart Rate Max: Recovery:

STRENGTH: UPPER BODY & BACK		STRENGTH: LEGS & ABS	
1:	Reps:	1:	Reps:
2:	Reps:	2:	Reps:
3:	Reps:	3:	Reps:
4:	Reps:	4:	Reps:
5:	Reps:	5:	Reps:

F O O D

Breakfast:

Lunch:

Dinner:

Snacks: Crap: Booze:

L I F E

Caring, connecting, committing:

How did you do?   ☐ Amazing   ☐ Not Bad   ☐ Shameful

Plans for tomorrow:

Tuesday _ | _ | _ |

How was your night?

Morning mood: Resting Heart Rate:

EXERCISE

CARDIO

Time and/or distance: Level: Heart Rate Max: Recovery:

STRENGTH: UPPER BODY & BACK		STRENGTH: LEGS & ABS	
1:	Reps:	1:	Reps:
2:	Reps:	2:	Reps:
3:	Reps:	3:	Reps:
4:	Reps:	4:	Reps:
5:	Reps:	5:	Reps:

FOOD

Breakfast:

Lunch:

Dinner:

Snacks: Crap: Booze:

LIFE

Caring, connecting, committing:

How did you do?   ☐ Amazing   ☐ Not Bad   ☐ Shameful

Plans for tomorrow:

Wednesday _ | _ | _ |

How was your night?

Morning mood: Resting Heart Rate:

EXERCISE

CARDIO

Time and/or distance: Level: Heart Rate Max: Recovery:

STRENGTH: UPPER BODY & BACK		STRENGTH: LEGS & ABS	
1:	Reps:	1:	Reps:
2:	Reps:	2:	Reps:
3:	Reps:	3:	Reps:
4:	Reps:	4:	Reps:
5:	Reps:	5:	Reps:

FOOD

Breakfast:

Lunch:

Dinner:

Snacks: Crap: Booze:

LIFE

Caring, connecting, committing:

How did you do?   ☐ Amazing   ☐ Not Bad   ☐ Shameful

Plans for tomorrow:

Thursday _ | | |

How was your night?

Morning mood: Resting Heart Rate:

EXERCISE

CARDIO

Time and/or distance: Level: Heart Rate Max: Recovery:

STRENGTH: UPPER BODY & BACK		STRENGTH: LEGS & ABS	
1:	Reps:	1:	Reps:
2:	Reps:	2:	Reps:
3:	Reps:	3:	Reps:
4:	Reps:	4:	Reps:
5:	Reps:	5:	Reps:

FOOD

Breakfast:

Lunch:

Dinner:

Snacks: Crap: Booze:

LIFE

Caring, connecting, committing:

How did you do?   ☐ Amazing   ☐ Not Bad   ☐ Shameful

Plans for tomorrow:

Friday _ | | |

How was your night?

Morning mood: Resting Heart Rate:

EXERCISE

CARDIO

Time and/or distance: Level: Heart Rate Max: Recovery:

STRENGTH: UPPER BODY & BACK		STRENGTH: LEGS & ABS	
1:	Reps:	1:	Reps:
2:	Reps:	2:	Reps:
3:	Reps:	3:	Reps:
4:	Reps:	4:	Reps:
5:	Reps:	5:	Reps:

FOOD

Breakfast:

Lunch:

Dinner:

Snacks: Crap: Booze:

LIFE

Caring, connecting, committing:

How did you do?   ☐ Amazing   ☐ Not Bad   ☐ Shameful

Plans for tomorrow:

Saturday ___ | ___ | ___

How was your night?

Morning mood: Resting Heart Rate:

EXERCISE

CARDIO

Time and/or distance: Level: Heart Rate Max: Recovery:

STRENGTH: UPPER BODY & BACK		STRENGTH: LEGS & ABS	
1:	Reps:	1:	Reps:
2:	Reps:	2:	Reps:
3:	Reps:	3:	Reps:
4:	Reps:	4:	Reps:
5:	Reps:	5:	Reps:

FOOD

Breakfast:

Lunch:

Dinner:

Snacks: Crap: Booze:

LIFE

Caring, connecting, committing:

How did you do?   ☐ Amazing ☐ Not Bad ☐ Shameful

Plans for tomorrow:

Sunday ___ | ___ | ___

How was your night?

Morning mood: Resting Heart Rate:

EXERCISE

CARDIO

Time and/or distance: Level: Heart Rate Max: Recovery:

STRENGTH: UPPER BODY & BACK		STRENGTH: LEGS & ABS	
1:	Reps:	1:	Reps:
2:	Reps:	2:	Reps:
3:	Reps:	3:	Reps:
4:	Reps:	4:	Reps:
5:	Reps:	5:	Reps:

FOOD

Breakfast:

Lunch:

Dinner:

Snacks: Crap: Booze:

LIFE

Caring, connecting, committing:

How did you do?   ☐ Amazing ☐ Not Bad ☐ Shameful

Plans for tomorrow:

26 week

Exercise & Diet Plan for the Week

	MONDAY	TUESDAY	WEDNESDAY	THURSDAY	FRIDAY	SATURDAY	SUNDAY
CARDIO							
WEIGHTS							

Weight at beginning of week: _____ Weight at end of week: _____

Goals for the week: _____

Ideas for caring, connecting, committing: _____

CHRIS SAYS: **CHECK YOUR RECOVERY RATE**

Harry and I seldom disagree, but I think your "recovery rate" is a much better indicator of what's going on in your body than your resting pulse. You compute it like this: Crank your heart rate up to, say, 80% or more of your max. Then slow way down, check your heart rate monitor, and start watching the second hand of your watch. At the first tick, time yourself for sixty seconds. Then check your heart rate. The difference is your recovery rate. Forty is great, but anything over twenty isn't bad. If your recovery rate is low, resolve to put in more "long and slow" time.

Monday ___ ___ ___

How was your night? _____

Morning mood: _____ Resting Heart Rate: _____

EXERCISE

CARDIO

Time and/or distance: _____ Level: _____ Heart Rate Max: _____ Recovery: _____

STRENGTH: UPPER BODY & BACK		**STRENGTH: LEGS & ABS**	
1:	Reps:	1:	Reps:
2:	Reps:	2:	Reps:
3:	Reps:	3:	Reps:
4:	Reps:	4:	Reps:
5:	Reps:	5:	Reps:

FOOD

Breakfast:

Lunch:

Dinner:

Snacks: _____ Crap: _____ Booze: _____

LIFE

Caring, connecting, committing:

How did you do?   ☐ Amazing   ☐ Not Bad   ☐ Shameful

Plans for tomorrow:

Tuesday ___ | ___ | ___

How was your night?

Morning mood: Resting Heart Rate:

E X E R C I S E

CARDIO

Time and/or distance: Level: Heart Rate Max: Recovery:

STRENGTH: UPPER BODY & BACK		STRENGTH: LEGS & ABS	
1:	Reps:	1:	Reps:
2:	Reps:	2:	Reps:
3:	Reps:	3:	Reps:
4:	Reps:	4:	Reps:
5:	Reps:	5:	Reps:

F O O D

Breakfast:

Lunch:

Dinner:

Snacks: Crap: Booze:

L I F E

Caring, connecting, committing:

How did you do? ☐ Amazing ☐ Not Bad ☐ Shameful

Plans for tomorrow:

Wednesday ___ | ___ | ___

How was your night?

Morning mood: Resting Heart Rate:

E X E R C I S E

CARDIO

Time and/or distance: Level: Heart Rate Max: Recovery:

STRENGTH: UPPER BODY & BACK		STRENGTH: LEGS & ABS	
1:	Reps:	1:	Reps:
2:	Reps:	2:	Reps:
3:	Reps:	3:	Reps:
4:	Reps:	4:	Reps:
5:	Reps:	5:	Reps:

F O O D

Breakfast:

Lunch:

Dinner:

Snacks: Crap: Booze:

L I F E

Caring, connecting, committing:

How did you do? ☐ Amazing ☐ Not Bad ☐ Shameful

Plans for tomorrow:

Thursday

How was your night?

Morning mood: Resting Heart Rate:

EXERCISE

CARDIO

Time and/or distance: Level: Heart Rate Max: Recovery:

STRENGTH: UPPER BODY & BACK		STRENGTH: LEGS & ABS	
1:	Reps:	1:	Reps:
2:	Reps:	2:	Reps:
3:	Reps:	3:	Reps:
4:	Reps:	4:	Reps:
5:	Reps:	5:	Reps:

FOOD

Breakfast:

Lunch:

Dinner:

Snacks: Crap: Booze:

LIFE

Caring, connecting, committing:

How did you do?   ☐ Amazing ☐ Not Bad ☐ Shameful

Plans for tomorrow:

Friday

How was your night?

Morning mood: Resting Heart Rate:

EXERCISE

CARDIO

Time and/or distance: Level: Heart Rate Max: Recovery:

STRENGTH: UPPER BODY & BACK		STRENGTH: LEGS & ABS	
1:	Reps:	1:	Reps:
2:	Reps:	2:	Reps:
3:	Reps:	3:	Reps:
4:	Reps:	4:	Reps:
5:	Reps:	5:	Reps:

FOOD

Breakfast:

Lunch:

Dinner:

Snacks: Crap: Booze:

LIFE

Caring, connecting, committing:

How did you do?   ☐ Amazing ☐ Not Bad ☐ Shameful

Plans for tomorrow:

Saturday __ | __ | __

How was your night?

Morning mood: Resting Heart Rate:

E X E R C I S E

CARDIO

Time and/or distance: Level: Heart Rate Max: Recovery:

STRENGTH: UPPER BODY & BACK		STRENGTH: LEGS & ABS	
1:	Reps:	1:	Reps:
2:	Reps:	2:	Reps:
3:	Reps:	3:	Reps:
4:	Reps:	4:	Reps:
5:	Reps:	5:	Reps:

F O O D

Breakfast:

Lunch.

Dinner:

Snacks: Crap: Booze:

L I F E

Caring, connecting, committing:

How did you do? ☐ Amazing ☐ Not Bad ☐ Shameful

Plans for tomorrow:

Sunday __ | __ | __

How was your night?

Morning mood: Resting Heart Rate:

E X E R C I S E

CARDIO

Time and/or distance: Level: Heart Rate Max: Recovery:

STRENGTH: UPPER BODY & BACK		STRENGTH: LEGS & ABS	
1:	Reps:	1:	Reps:
2:	Reps:	2:	Reps:
3:	Reps:	3:	Reps:
4:	Reps:	4:	Reps:
5:	Reps:	5:	Reps:

F O O D

Breakfast:

Lunch:

Dinner:

Snacks: Crap: Booze:

L I F E

Caring, connecting, committing:

How did you do? ☐ Amazing ☐ Not Bad ☐ Shameful

Plans for tomorrow:

Exercise & Diet Plan for the Week

	MONDAY	TUESDAY	WEDNESDAY	THURSDAY	FRIDAY	SATURDAY	SUNDAY
CARDIO							
WEIGHTS							

Weight at beginning of week: _____ Weight at end of week: _____

Goals for the week: _____

Ideas for caring, connecting, committing: _____

HARRY SAYS: **EAT FOR ONE, NOT FOUR**

Try this experiment, just for fun. Go to your local pancake house and order a special breakfast—you know, the kind that comes with three large pancakes, two eggs, sausage, bacon, home fries, and toast. The plate will essentially be the size of a serving platter. Don't start eating! Instead, divide the meal into rational portion sizes. Then invite another three people over to share your breakfast.

Monday ___|___|___

How was your night?

Morning mood: _____ Resting Heart Rate: _____

E X E R C I S E

CARDIO

Time and/or distance: _____ Level: _____ Heart Rate Max: _____ Recovery: _____

STRENGTH: UPPER BODY & BACK		**STRENGTH: LEGS & ABS**	
1:	Reps:	1:	Reps:
2:	Reps:	2:	Reps:
3:	Reps:	3:	Reps:
4:	Reps:	4:	Reps:
5:	Reps:	5:	Reps:

F O O D

Breakfast:

Lunch:

Dinner:

Snacks: _____ Crap: _____ Booze: _____

L I F E

Caring, connecting, committing:

How did you do? ☐ Amazing ☐ Not Bad ☐ Shameful

Plans for tomorrow:

Tuesday ☐ ☐ ☐

How was your night?

Morning mood: _____ Resting Heart Rate: _____

EXERCISE

CARDIO

Time and/or distance: _____ Level: _____ Heart Rate Max: _____ Recovery: _____

STRENGTH: UPPER BODY & BACK		STRENGTH: LEGS & ABS	
1:	Reps:	1:	Reps:
2:	Reps:	2:	Reps:
3:	Reps:	3:	Reps:
4:	Reps:	4:	Reps:
5:	Reps:	5:	Reps:

FOOD

Breakfast:

Lunch:

Dinner:

Snacks: _____ Crap: _____ Booze: _____

LIFE

Caring, connecting, committing:

How did you do? ☐ Amazing ☐ Not Bad ☐ Shameful

Plans for tomorrow:

Wednesday ☐ ☐

How was your night?

Morning mood: _____ Resting Heart Rate: _____

EXERCISE

CARDIO

Time and/or distance: _____ Level: _____ Heart Rate Max: _____ Recovery: _____

STRENGTH: UPPER BODY & BACK		STRENGTH: LEGS & ABS	
1:	Reps:	1:	Reps:
2:	Reps:	2:	Reps:
3:	Reps:	3:	Reps:
4:	Reps:	4:	Reps:
5:	Reps:	5:	Reps:

FOOD

Breakfast:

Lunch:

Dinner:

Snacks: _____ Crap: _____ Booze: _____

LIFE

Caring, connecting, committing:

How did you do? ☐ Amazing ☐ Not Bad ☐ Shameful

Plans for tomorrow:

Thursday____ | | |

How was your night?

Morning mood: Resting Heart Rate:

E X E R C I S E

CARDIO

Time and/or distance: Level: Heart Rate Max: Recovery:

STRENGTH: UPPER BODY & BACK		STRENGTH: LEGS & ABS	
1:	Reps:	1:	Reps:
2:	Reps:	2:	Reps:
3:	Reps:	3:	Reps:
4:	Reps:	4:	Reps:
5:	Reps:	5:	Reps:

F O O D

Breakfast:

Lunch:

Dinner:

Snacks: Crap: Booze:

L I F E

Caring, connecting, committing:

How did you do?   ☐ Amazing   ☐ Not Bad   ☐ Shameful

Plans for tomorrow:

Friday____ | | |

How was your night?

Morning mood: Resting Heart Rate:

E X E R C I S E

CARDIO

Time and/or distance: Level: Heart Rate Max: Recovery:

STRENGTH: UPPER BODY & BACK		STRENGTH: LEGS & ABS	
1:	Reps:	1:	Reps:
2:	Reps:	2:	Reps:
3:	Reps:	3:	Reps:
4:	Reps:	4:	Reps:
5:	Reps:	5:	Reps:

F O O D

Breakfast:

Lunch:

Dinner:

Snacks: Crap: Booze:

L I F E

Caring, connecting, committing:

How did you do?   ☐ Amazing   ☐ Not Bad   ☐ Shameful

Plans for tomorrow:

Saturday___|___|___|

How was your night?

Morning mood: Resting Heart Rate:

E X E R C I S E

CARDIO

Time and/or distance: Level: Heart Rate Max: Recovery:

STRENGTH: UPPER BODY & BACK		STRENGTH: LEGS & ABS	
1:	Reps:	1:	Reps:
2:	Reps:	2:	Reps:
3:	Reps:	3:	Reps:
4:	Reps:	4:	Reps:
5:	Reps:	5:	Reps:

F O O D

Breakfast:

Lunch:

Dinner:

Snacks: Crap: Booze:

L I F E

Caring, connecting, committing:

How did you do?   ☐ Amazing ☐ Not Bad ☐ Shameful

Plans for tomorrow:

Sunday___|___|___|

How was your night?

Morning mood: Resting Heart Rate:

E X E R C I S E

CARDIO

Time and/or distance: Level: Heart Rate Max: Recovery:

STRENGTH: UPPER BODY & BACK		STRENGTH: LEGS & ABS	
1:	Reps:	1:	Reps:
2:	Reps:	2:	Reps:
3:	Reps:	3:	Reps:
4:	Reps:	4:	Reps:
5:	Reps:	5:	Reps:

F O O D

Breakfast:

Lunch:

Dinner:

Snacks: Crap: Booze:

L I F E

Caring, connecting, committing:

How did you do?   ☐ Amazing ☐ Not Bad ☐ Shameful

Plans for tomorrow:

28 week | Exercise & Diet Plan for the Week

	MONDAY	TUESDAY	WEDNESDAY	THURSDAY	FRIDAY	SATURDAY	SUNDAY
CARDIO							
WEIGHTS							

Weight at beginning of week: _____   Weight at end of week: _____

Goals for the week: _____

Ideas for caring, connecting, committing: _____

CHRIS SAYS: GET SOME DECENT DUDS

Back in my early days of going to the gym, I concluded that I looked stupid enough without dressing like an idiot or a loser. So I bought some semi-modern dress, since only the very young and beautiful can afford to be heedless about how they look. This is not, however, an excuse not to go to the gym. Better to go in Auntie's bloomers and snood than to stay home. But eventually get some nice workout clothes. And good sneakers. It'll keep your spirits up.

Monday ___ | | |

How was your night? _____
Morning mood: _____   Resting Heart Rate: _____

EXERCISE

CARDIO

Time and/or distance: _____   Level: _____   Heart Rate Max: _____   Recovery: _____

STRENGTH: UPPER BODY & BACK		STRENGTH: LEGS & ABS	
1:	Reps:	1:	Reps:
2:	Reps:	2:	Reps:
3:	Reps:	3:	Reps:
4:	Reps:	4:	Reps:
5:	Reps:	5:	Reps:

FOOD

Breakfast:

Lunch:

Dinner:

Snacks: _____   Crap: _____   Booze: _____

LIFE

Caring, connecting, committing:

How did you do?   ☐ Amazing   ☐ Not Bad   ☐ Shameful

Plans for tomorrow:

Tuesday ___ | ___ | ___

How was your night?

Morning mood: Resting Heart Rate:

EXERCISE

CARDIO

Time and/or distance: Level: Heart Rate Max: Recovery:

STRENGTH: UPPER BODY & BACK		STRENGTH: LEGS & ABS	
1:	Reps:	1:	Reps:
2:	Reps:	2:	Reps:
3:	Reps:	3:	Reps:
4:	Reps:	4:	Reps:
5:	Reps:	5:	Reps:

FOOD

Breakfast:

Lunch:

Dinner:

Snacks: Crap: Booze:

LIFE

Caring, connecting, committing:

How did you do? ☐ Amazing ☐ Not Bad ☐ Shameful

Plans for tomorrow:

Wednesday ___ | ___ | ___

How was your night?

Morning mood: Resting Heart Rate:

EXERCISE

CARDIO

Time and/or distance: Level: Heart Rate Max: Recovery:

STRENGTH: UPPER BODY & BACK		STRENGTH: LEGS & ABS	
1:	Reps:	1:	Reps:
2:	Reps:	2:	Reps:
3:	Reps:	3:	Reps:
4:	Reps:	4:	Reps:
5:	Reps:	5:	Reps:

FOOD

Breakfast:

Lunch:

Dinner:

Snacks: Crap: Booze:

LIFE

Caring, connecting, committing:

How did you do? ☐ Amazing ☐ Not Bad ☐ Shameful

Plans for tomorrow:

Thursday␣␣|␣|␣|

How was your night?

Morning mood:⠀⠀⠀⠀⠀Resting Heart Rate:

E X E R C I S E

CARDIO

Time and/or distance:⠀⠀Level:⠀⠀⠀Heart Rate Max:⠀⠀Recovery:

STRENGTH: UPPER BODY & BACK		STRENGTH: LEGS & ABS	
1:	Reps:	1:	Reps:
2:	Reps:	2:	Reps:
3:	Reps:	3:	Reps:
4:	Reps:	4:	Reps:
5:	Reps:	5:	Reps:

F O O D

Breakfast:

Lunch:

Dinner:

Snacks:⠀⠀⠀⠀⠀Crap:⠀⠀⠀⠀⠀Booze:

L I F E

Caring, connecting, committing:

How did you do?⠀☐ Amazing⠀☐ Not Bad⠀☐ Shameful

Plans for tomorrow:

Friday␣␣|␣|␣|

How was your night?

Morning mood:⠀⠀⠀⠀⠀Resting Heart Rate:

E X E R C I S E

CARDIO

Time and/or distance:⠀⠀Level:⠀⠀⠀Heart Rate Max:⠀⠀Recovery:

STRENGTH: UPPER BODY & BACK		STRENGTH: LEGS & ABS	
1:	Reps:	1:	Reps:
2:	Reps:	2:	Reps:
3:	Reps:	3:	Reps:
4:	Reps:	4:	Reps:
5:	Reps:	5:	Reps:

F O O D

Breakfast:

Lunch:

Dinner:

Snacks:⠀⠀⠀⠀⠀Crap:⠀⠀⠀⠀⠀Booze:

L I F E

Caring, connecting, committing:

How did you do?⠀☐ Amazing⠀☐ Not Bad⠀☐ Shameful

Plans for tomorrow:

Saturday____|__|__|

How was your night?	
Morning mood:	Resting Heart Rate:

EXERCISE

CARDIO

Time and/or distance:	Level:	Heart Rate Max:	Recovery:

STRENGTH: UPPER BODY & BACK		STRENGTH: LEGS & ABS	
1:	Reps:	1:	Reps:
2:	Reps:	2:	Reps:
3:	Reps:	3:	Reps:
4:	Reps:	4:	Reps:
5:	Reps:	5:	Reps:

FOOD

Breakfast:

Lunch:

Dinner:

Snacks:	Crap:	Booze:

LIFE

Caring, connecting, committing:

How did you do? ☐ Amazing ☐ Not Bad ☐ Shameful

Plans for tomorrow:

Sunday____|__|__|

How was your night?	
Morning mood:	Resting Heart Rate:

EXERCISE

CARDIO

Time and/or distance:	Level:	Heart Rate Max:	Recovery:

STRENGTH: UPPER BODY & BACK		STRENGTH: LEGS & ABS	
1:	Reps:	1:	Reps:
2:	Reps:	2:	Reps:
3:	Reps:	3:	Reps:
4:	Reps:	4:	Reps:
5:	Reps:	5:	Reps:

FOOD

Breakfast:

Lunch:

Dinner:

Snacks:	Crap:	Booze:

LIFE

Caring, connecting, committing:

How did you do? ☐ Amazing ☐ Not Bad ☐ Shameful

Plans for tomorrow:

29 week

Exercise & Diet Plan for the Week

	MONDAY	TUESDAY	WEDNESDAY	THURSDAY	FRIDAY	SATURDAY	SUNDAY
CARDIO							
WEIGHTS							

Weight at beginning of week: _____ Weight at end of week: _____

Goals for the week: _____

Ideas for caring, connecting, committing: _____

HARRY SAYS: **WORK YOUR BODY**

Since blood is redirected not only to muscles you're working but to that whole area of the body, it makes sense to do all your leg exercises together, your arm exercises together, and your core (crunch) exercises together. That said, you can do the three body areas in any order you want. Mix it up so you don't get bored.

Monday___|___|___|

How was your night? _____

Morning mood: _____ Resting Heart Rate: _____

E X E R C I S E

CARDIO

Time and/or distance: _____ Level: _____ Heart Rate Max: _____ Recovery: _____

STRENGTH: UPPER BODY & BACK		**STRENGTH: LEGS & ABS**	
1:	Reps:	1:	Reps:
2:	Reps:	2:	Reps:
3:	Reps:	3:	Reps:
4:	Reps:	4:	Reps:
5:	Reps:	5:	Reps:

F O O D

Breakfast:

Lunch:

Dinner:

Snacks: _____ Crap: _____ Booze: _____

L I F E

Caring, connecting, committing:

How did you do? ☐ Amazing ☐ Not Bad ☐ Shameful

Plans for tomorrow:

Tuesday _|_ |_ |_

How was your night?

Morning mood: Resting Heart Rate:

EXERCISE

CARDIO

Time and/or distance: Level: Heart Rate Max: Recovery:

STRENGTH: UPPER BODY & BACK		STRENGTH: LEGS & ABS	
1:	Reps:	1:	Reps:
2:	Reps:	2:	Reps:
3:	Reps:	3:	Reps:
4:	Reps:	4:	Reps:
5:	Reps:	5:	Reps:

FOOD

Breakfast:

Lunch:

Dinner:

Snacks: Crap: Booze:

LIFE

Caring, connecting, committing:

How did you do?   ☐ Amazing   ☐ Not Bad   ☐ Shameful

Plans for tomorrow:

Wednesday _|_ |_ |_

How was your night?

Morning mood: Resting Heart Rate:

EXERCISE

CARDIO

Time and/or distance: Level: Heart Rate Max: Recovery:

STRENGTH: UPPER BODY & BACK		STRENGTH: LEGS & ABS	
1:	Reps:	1:	Reps:
2:	Reps:	2:	Reps:
3:	Reps:	3:	Reps:
4:	Reps:	4:	Reps:
5:	Reps:	5:	Reps:

FOOD

Breakfast:

Lunch:

Dinner:

Snacks: Crap: Booze:

LIFE

Caring, connecting, committing:

How did you do?   ☐ Amazing   ☐ Not Bad   ☐ Shameful

Plans for tomorrow:

Thursday␣␣␣

How was your night?

Morning mood: Resting Heart Rate:

EXERCISE

CARDIO

Time and/or distance: Level: Heart Rate Max: Recovery:

STRENGTH: UPPER BODY & BACK		STRENGTH: LEGS & ABS	
1:	Reps:	1:	Reps:
2:	Reps:	2:	Reps:
3:	Reps:	3:	Reps:
4:	Reps:	4:	Reps:
5:	Reps:	5:	Reps:

FOOD

Breakfast:

Lunch:

Dinner:

Snacks: Crap: Booze:

LIFE

Caring, connecting, committing:

How did you do?   ☐ Amazing ☐ Not Bad ☐ Shameful

Plans for tomorrow:

Friday␣␣␣

How was your night?

Morning mood: Resting Heart Rate:

EXERCISE

CARDIO

Time and/or distance: Level: Heart Rate Max: Recovery:

STRENGTH: UPPER BODY & BACK		STRENGTH: LEGS & ABS	
1:	Reps:	1:	Reps:
2:	Reps:	2:	Reps:
3:	Reps:	3:	Reps:
4:	Reps:	4:	Reps:
5:	Reps:	5:	Reps:

FOOD

Breakfast:

Lunch:

Dinner:

Snacks: Crap: Booze:

LIFE

Caring, connecting, committing:

How did you do?   ☐ Amazing ☐ Not Bad ☐ Shameful

Plans for tomorrow:

Saturday___|__|__|

How was your night?

Morning mood: Resting Heart Rate:

E X E R C I S E

CARDIO

Time and/or distance: Level: Heart Rate Max: Recovery:

STRENGTH: UPPER BODY & BACK		STRENGTH: LEGS & ABS	
1:	Reps:	1:	Reps:
2:	Reps:	2:	Reps:
3:	Reps:	3:	Reps:
4:	Reps:	4:	Reps:
5:	Reps:	5:	Reps:

F O O D

Breakfast:

Lunch:

Dinner:

Snacks: Crap: Booze:

L I F E

Caring, connecting, committing:

How did you do?   ☐ Amazing ☐ Not Bad ☐ Shameful

Plans for tomorrow:

Sunday___|__|__|

How was your night?

Morning mood: Resting Heart Rate:

E X E R C I S E

CARDIO

Time and/or distance: Level: Heart Rate Max: Recovery:

STRENGTH: UPPER BODY & BACK		STRENGTH: LEGS & ABS	
1:	Reps:	1:	Reps:
2:	Reps:	2:	Reps:
3:	Reps:	3:	Reps:
4:	Reps:	4:	Reps:
5:	Reps:	5:	Reps:

F O O D

Breakfast:

Lunch:

Dinner:

Snacks: Crap: Booze:

L I F E

Caring, connecting, committing:

How did you do?   ☐ Amazing ☐ Not Bad ☐ Shameful

Plans for tomorrow:

Exercise & Diet Plan for the Week

	MONDAY	TUESDAY	WEDNESDAY	THURSDAY	FRIDAY	SATURDAY	SUNDAY
CARDIO							
WEIGHTS							

Weight at beginning of week: Weight at end of week:

Goals for the week:

Ideas for caring, connecting, committing:

CHRIS SAYS: GO OUTDOORS

You may not believe this yet, but some people get addicted to the gym. Well, that's great, but you have to get outside, too. Ride a *real* bike. Go for a swim in the ocean. Climb a mountain. The change will keep you going, and make it all the more fun. Hey, you're not a gerbil running on a wheel. And you shouldn't be a gym rat either.

Monday | | |

How was your night?

Morning mood: Resting Heart Rate:

E X E R C I S E

CARDIO

Time and/or distance: Level: Heart Rate Max: Recovery:

STRENGTH: UPPER BODY & BACK		STRENGTH: LEGS & ABS	
1:	Reps:	1:	Reps:
2:	Reps:	2:	Reps:
3:	Reps:	3:	Reps:
4:	Reps:	4:	Reps:
5:	Reps:	5:	Reps:

F O O D

Breakfast:

Lunch:

Dinner:

Snacks: Crap: Booze:

L I F E

Caring, connecting, committing:

How did you do? ☐ Amazing ☐ Not Bad ☐ Shameful

Plans for tomorrow:

Tuesday | | |

How was your night?

Morning mood: Resting Heart Rate:

EXERCISE

CARDIO

Time and/or distance: Level: Heart Rate Max: Recovery:

STRENGTH: UPPER BODY & BACK		STRENGTH: LEGS & ABS	
1:	Reps:	1:	Reps:
2:	Reps:	2:	Reps:
3:	Reps:	3:	Reps:
4:	Reps:	4:	Reps:
5:	Reps:	5:	Reps:

FOOD

Breakfast:

Lunch:

Dinner:

Snacks: Crap: Booze:

LIFE

Caring, connecting, committing:

How did you do?   ☐ Amazing ☐ Not Bad ☐ Shameful

Plans for tomorrow:

Wednesday | | |

How was your night?

Morning mood: Resting Heart Rate:

EXERCISE

CARDIO

Time and/or distance: Level: Heart Rate Max: Recovery:

STRENGTH: UPPER BODY & BACK		STRENGTH: LEGS & ABS	
1:	Reps:	1:	Reps:
2:	Reps:	2:	Reps:
3:	Reps:	3:	Reps:
4:	Reps:	4:	Reps:
5:	Reps:	5:	Reps:

FOOD

Breakfast:

Lunch:

Dinner:

Snacks: Crap: Booze:

LIFE

Caring, connecting, committing:

How did you do?   ☐ Amazing ☐ Not Bad ☐ Shameful

Plans for tomorrow:

Thursday___|___|___

How was your night?

Morning mood: Resting Heart Rate:

E X E R C I S E

CARDIO

Time and/or distance: Level: Heart Rate Max: Recovery:

STRENGTH: UPPER BODY & BACK		STRENGTH: LEGS & ABS	
1:	Reps:	1:	Reps:
2:	Reps:	2:	Reps:
3:	Reps:	3:	Reps:
4:	Reps:	4:	Reps:
5:	Reps:	5:	Reps:

F O O D

Breakfast:

Lunch:

Dinner:

Snacks: Crap: Booze:

L I F E

Caring, connecting, committing:

How did you do?   ☐ Amazing   ☐ Not Bad   ☐ Shameful

Plans for tomorrow:

Friday___|___|___

How was your night?

Morning mood: Resting Heart Rate:

E X E R C I S E

CARDIO

Time and/or distance: Level: Heart Rate Max: Recovery:

STRENGTH: UPPER BODY & BACK		STRENGTH: LEGS & ABS	
1:	Reps:	1:	Reps:
2:	Reps:	2:	Reps:
3:	Reps:	3:	Reps:
4:	Reps:	4:	Reps:
5:	Reps:	5:	Reps:

F O O D

Breakfast:

Lunch:

Dinner:

Snacks: Crap: Booze:

L I F E

Caring, connecting, committing:

How did you do?   ☐ Amazing   ☐ Not Bad   ☐ Shameful

Plans for tomorrow:

Saturday_|_|_

How was your night?

Morning mood: Resting Heart Rate:

E X E R C I S E

CARDIO

Time and/or distance: Level: Heart Rate Max: Recovery:

STRENGTH: UPPER BODY & BACK		STRENGTH: LEGS & ABS	
1:	Reps:	1:	Reps:
2:	Reps:	2:	Reps:
3:	Reps:	3:	Reps:
4:	Reps:	4:	Reps:
5:	Reps:	5:	Reps:

F O O D

Breakfast:

Lunch:

Dinner:

Snacks: Crap: Booze:

L I F E

Caring, connecting, committing:

How did you do?   ☐ Amazing ☐ Not Bad ☐ Shameful

Plans for tomorrow:

Sunday_|_|_

How was your night?

Morning mood: Resting Heart Rate:

E X E R C I S E

CARDIO

Time and/or distance: Level: Heart Rate Max: Recovery:

STRENGTH: UPPER BODY & BACK		STRENGTH: LEGS & ABS	
1:	Reps:	1:	Reps:
2:	Reps:	2:	Reps:
3:	Reps:	3:	Reps:
4:	Reps:	4:	Reps:
5:	Reps:	5:	Reps:

F O O D

Breakfast:

Lunch:

Dinner:

Snacks: Crap: Booze:

L I F E

Caring, connecting, committing:

How did you do?   ☐ Amazing ☐ Not Bad ☐ Shameful

Plans for tomorrow:

31 week Exercise & Diet Plan for the Week

	MONDAY	TUESDAY	WEDNESDAY	THURSDAY	FRIDAY	SATURDAY	SUNDAY
CARDIO							
WEIGHTS							

Weight at beginning of week: _____   Weight at end of week: _____

Goals for the week: _____

Ideas for caring, connecting, committing: _____

HARRY SAYS: WARM DOWN

Even if you're pressed for time, don't abruptly stop exercising, particularly if you've been working at 75–80% of your max. If you do, your blood flow will rapidly shift over to the areas of your body that have been dormant—your liver, your intestines, and so on. And you may find that your muscles, deprived of that blood flow, will start complaining. To keep yourself from getting stiff, just move gently for a few minutes after you stop exercising. But no need to taper off if you've been having a "long and slow" exercise day.

Monday ⎵ ⎵ ⎵

How was your night? _____

Morning mood: _____   Resting Heart Rate: _____

EXERCISE

CARDIO

Time and/or distance: _____   Level: _____   Heart Rate Max: _____   Recovery: _____

STRENGTH: UPPER BODY & BACK		STRENGTH: LEGS & ABS	
1:	Reps:	1:	Reps:
2:	Reps:	2:	Reps:
3:	Reps:	3:	Reps:
4:	Reps:	4:	Reps:
5:	Reps:	5:	Reps:

FOOD

Breakfast:

Lunch:

Dinner:

Snacks: _____   Crap: _____   Booze: _____

LIFE

Caring, connecting, committing:

How did you do?   ☐ Amazing   ☐ Not Bad   ☐ Shameful

Plans for tomorrow:

Tuesday␣␣␣

How was your night?

Morning mood: Resting Heart Rate:

EXERCISE

CARDIO

Time and/or distance: Level: Heart Rate Max: Recovery:

STRENGTH: UPPER BODY & BACK		STRENGTH: LEGS & ABS	
1:	Reps:	1:	Reps:
2:	Reps:	2:	Reps:
3:	Reps:	3:	Reps:
4:	Reps:	4:	Reps:
5:	Reps:	5:	Reps:

FOOD

Breakfast:

Lunch:

Dinner:

Snacks: Crap: Booze:

LIFE

Caring, connecting, committing:

How did you do? ☐ Amazing ☐ Not Bad ☐ Shameful

Plans for tomorrow:

Wednesday␣␣␣

How was your night?

Morning mood: Resting Heart Rate:

EXERCISE

CARDIO

Time and/or distance: Level: Heart Rate Max: Recovery:

STRENGTH: UPPER BODY & BACK		STRENGTH: LEGS & ABS	
1:	Reps:	1:	Reps:
2:	Reps:	2:	Reps:
3:	Reps:	3:	Reps:
4:	Reps:	4:	Reps:
5:	Reps:	5:	Reps:

FOOD

Breakfast:

Lunch:

Dinner:

Snacks: Crap: Booze:

LIFE

Caring, connecting, committing:

How did you do? ☐ Amazing ☐ Not Bad ☐ Shameful

Plans for tomorrow:

Thursday __ | | |

How was your night?

Morning mood: Resting Heart Rate:

EXERCISE

CARDIO

Time and/or distance: Level: Heart Rate Max: Recovery:

STRENGTH: UPPER BODY & BACK		STRENGTH: LEGS & ABS	
1:	Reps:	1:	Reps:
2:	Reps:	2:	Reps:
3:	Reps:	3:	Reps:
4:	Reps:	4:	Reps:
5:	Reps:	5:	Reps:

FOOD

Breakfast:

Lunch:

Dinner:

Snacks: Crap: Booze:

LIFE

Caring, connecting, committing:

How did you do? ☐ Amazing ☐ Not Bad ☐ Shameful

Plans for tomorrow:

Friday __ | | |

How was your night?

Morning mood: Resting Heart Rate:

EXERCISE

CARDIO

Time and/or distance: Level: Heart Rate Max: Recovery:

STRENGTH: UPPER BODY & BACK		STRENGTH: LEGS & ABS	
1:	Reps:	1:	Reps:
2:	Reps:	2:	Reps:
3:	Reps:	3:	Reps:
4:	Reps:	4:	Reps:
5:	Reps:	5:	Reps:

FOOD

Breakfast:

Lunch:

Dinner:

Snacks: Crap: Booze:

LIFE

Caring, connecting, committing:

How did you do? ☐ Amazing ☐ Not Bad ☐ Shameful

Plans for tomorrow:

Saturday ☐ ☐ ☐

How was your night?

Morning mood: Resting Heart Rate:

EXERCISE

CARDIO

Time and/or distance: Level: Heart Rate Max: Recovery:

STRENGTH: UPPER BODY & BACK		STRENGTH: LEGS & ABS	
1:	Reps:	1:	Reps:
2:	Reps:	2:	Reps:
3:	Reps:	3:	Reps:
4:	Reps:	4:	Reps:
5:	Reps:	5:	Reps:

FOOD

Breakfast:

Lunch.

Dinner:

Snacks: Crap: Booze:

LIFE

Caring, connecting, committing:

How did you do?   ☐ Amazing   ☐ Not Bad   ☐ Shameful

Plans for tomorrow:

Sunday ☐ ☐ ☐

How was your night?

Morning mood: Resting Heart Rate:

EXERCISE

CARDIO

Time and/or distance: Level: Heart Rate Max: Recovery:

STRENGTH: UPPER BODY & BACK		STRENGTH: LEGS & ABS	
1:	Reps:	1:	Reps:
2:	Reps:	2:	Reps:
3:	Reps:	3:	Reps:
4:	Reps:	4:	Reps:
5:	Reps:	5:	Reps:

FOOD

Breakfast:

Lunch:

Dinner:

Snacks: Crap: Booze:

LIFE

Caring, connecting, committing:

How did you do?   ☐ Amazing   ☐ Not Bad   ☐ Shameful

Plans for tomorrow:

32 week

Exercise & Diet Plan for the Week

	MONDAY	TUESDAY	WEDNESDAY	THURSDAY	FRIDAY	SATURDAY	SUNDAY
CARDIO							
WEIGHTS							

Weight at beginning of week: Weight at end of week:

Goals for the week:

Ideas for caring, connecting, committing:

CHRIS SAYS: LOOK IN THE MIRROR

I know, you may not like what you see, but checking yourself in the mirror (and gyms are full of them) makes it easier to tell if you're doing something right (or wrong). If you look hideous—and we all look hideous in the early stages—you'll be motivated to look less so. If you look okay, it will keep you going . . . part of the payoff. You're entitled to that.

Monday ___ ___

How was your night?

Morning mood: Resting Heart Rate:

E X E R C I S E

CARDIO

Time and/or distance: Level: Heart Rate Max: Recovery:

STRENGTH: UPPER BODY & BACK		**STRENGTH: LEGS & ABS**	
1:	Reps:	1:	Reps:
2:	Reps:	2:	Reps:
3:	Reps:	3:	Reps:
4:	Reps:	4:	Reps:
5:	Reps:	5:	Reps:

F O O D

Breakfast:

Lunch:

Dinner:

Snacks: Crap: Booze:

L I F E

Caring, connecting, committing:

How did you do? ☐ Amazing ☐ Not Bad ☐ Shameful

Plans for tomorrow:

Tuesday____|__|__|

How was your night?

Morning mood: Resting Heart Rate:

EXERCISE

CARDIO

Time and/or distance: Level: Heart Rate Max: Recovery:

STRENGTH: UPPER BODY & BACK		STRENGTH: LEGS & ABS	
1:	Reps:	1:	Reps:
2:	Reps:	2:	Reps:
3:	Reps:	3:	Reps:
4:	Reps:	4:	Reps:
5:	Reps:	5:	Reps:

FOOD

Breakfast:

Lunch:

Dinner:

Snacks: Crap: Booze:

LIFE

Caring, connecting, committing:

How did you do?   ☐ Amazing ☐ Not Bad ☐ Shameful

Plans for tomorrow:

Wednesday____|__|__|

How was your night?

Morning mood: Resting Heart Rate:

EXERCISE

CARDIO

Time and/or distance: Level: Heart Rate Max: Recovery:

STRENGTH: UPPER BODY & BACK		STRENGTH: LEGS & ABS	
1:	Reps:	1:	Reps:
2:	Reps:	2:	Reps:
3:	Reps:	3:	Reps:
4:	Reps:	4:	Reps:
5:	Reps:	5:	Reps:

FOOD

Breakfast:

Lunch:

Dinner:

Snacks: Crap: Booze:

LIFE

Caring, connecting, committing:

How did you do?   ☐ Amazing ☐ Not Bad ☐ Shameful

Plans for tomorrow:

Thursday___|___|___|

How was your night?

Morning mood: Resting Heart Rate:

EXERCISE

CARDIO

Time and/or distance: Level: Heart Rate Max: Recovery:

STRENGTH: UPPER BODY & BACK		STRENGTH: LEGS & ABS	
1:	Reps:	1:	Reps:
2:	Reps:	2:	Reps:
3:	Reps:	3:	Reps:
4:	Reps:	4:	Reps:
5:	Reps:	5:	Reps:

FOOD

Breakfast:

Lunch:

Dinner:

Snacks: Crap: Booze:

LIFE

Caring, connecting, committing:

How did you do?   ☐ Amazing   ☐ Not Bad   ☐ Shameful

Plans for tomorrow:

Friday___|___|___|

How was your night?

Morning mood: Resting Heart Rate:

EXERCISE

CARDIO

Time and/or distance: Level: Heart Rate Max: Recovery:

STRENGTH: UPPER BODY & BACK		STRENGTH: LEGS & ABS	
1:	Reps:	1:	Reps:
2:	Reps:	2:	Reps:
3:	Reps:	3:	Reps:
4:	Reps:	4:	Reps:
5:	Reps:	5:	Reps:

FOOD

Breakfast:

Lunch:

Dinner:

Snacks: Crap: Booze:

LIFE

Caring, connecting, committing:

How did you do?   ☐ Amazing   ☐ Not Bad   ☐ Shameful

Plans for tomorrow:

Saturday __|__|__

How was your night?

Morning mood: Resting Heart Rate:

EXERCISE

CARDIO

Time and/or distance: Level: Heart Rate Max: Recovery:

STRENGTH: UPPER BODY & BACK		STRENGTH: LEGS & ABS	
1:	Reps:	1:	Reps:
2:	Reps:	2:	Reps:
3:	Reps:	3:	Reps:
4:	Reps:	4:	Reps:
5:	Reps:	5:	Reps:

FOOD

Breakfast:

Lunch:

Dinner:

Snacks: Crap: Booze:

LIFE

Caring, connecting, committing:

How did you do?   ☐ Amazing ☐ Not Bad ☐ Shameful

Plans for tomorrow:

Sunday __|__|__

How was your night?

Morning mood: Resting Heart Rate:

EXERCISE

CARDIO

Time and/or distance: Level: Heart Rate Max: Recovery:

STRENGTH: UPPER BODY & BACK		STRENGTH: LEGS & ABS	
1:	Reps:	1:	Reps:
2:	Reps:	2:	Reps:
3:	Reps:	3:	Reps:
4:	Reps:	4:	Reps:
5:	Reps:	5:	Reps:

FOOD

Breakfast:

Lunch:

Dinner:

Snacks: Crap: Booze:

LIFE

Caring, connecting, committing:

How did you do?   ☐ Amazing ☐ Not Bad ☐ Shameful

Plans for tomorrow:

Exercise & Diet Plan for the Week

	MONDAY	TUESDAY	WEDNESDAY	THURSDAY	FRIDAY	SATURDAY	SUNDAY
CARDIO							
WEIGHTS							

Weight at beginning of week: _____ Weight at end of week: _____

Goals for the week: _____

Ideas for caring, connecting, committing: _____

HARRY SAYS: *PRE*-HYDRATE

Drinking a bottle of water at the gym after you've had a few cups of coffee (or just rolled out of bed) does you no good. Your level of hydration when you walk in the door is all that counts. So, toss down a tall glass of water the moment you wake up. And then chug a glass of water whenever you think of it. Have some fun: Can you get the whole glass down in one breath? (Hint: It's easier if the water's at room temperature.) Don't be shy about exercising if you haven't had three or four glasses of water, just notice how much better you feel on the days you do!

Monday | | |

How was your night? _____

Morning mood: _____ **Resting Heart Rate:** _____

EXERCISE

CARDIO

Time and/or distance: _____ Level: _____ Heart Rate Max: _____ Recovery: _____

STRENGTH: UPPER BODY & BACK		**STRENGTH: LEGS & ABS**	
1:	Reps:	1:	Reps:
2:	Reps:	2:	Reps:
3:	Reps:	3:	Reps:
4:	Reps:	4:	Reps:
5:	Reps:	5:	Reps:

FOOD

Breakfast: _____

Lunch: _____

Dinner: _____

Snacks: _____ Crap: _____ Booze: _____

LIFE

Caring, connecting, committing: _____

How did you do? ☐ Amazing ☐ Not Bad ☐ Shameful

Plans for tomorrow: _____

Tuesday ☐ ☐ ☐

How was your night?

Morning mood: Resting Heart Rate:

EXERCISE

CARDIO

Time and/or distance: Level: Heart Rate Max: Recovery:

STRENGTH: UPPER BODY & BACK		STRENGTH: LEGS & ABS	
1:	Reps:	1:	Reps:
2:	Reps:	2:	Reps:
3:	Reps:	3:	Reps:
4:	Reps:	4:	Reps:
5:	Reps:	5:	Reps:

FOOD

Breakfast:

Lunch:

Dinner:

Snacks: Crap: Booze:

LIFE

Caring, connecting, committing:

How did you do?   ☐ Amazing   ☐ Not Bad   ☐ Shameful

Plans for tomorrow:

Wednesday ☐ ☐ ☐

How was your night?

Morning mood: Resting Heart Rate:

EXERCISE

CARDIO

Time and/or distance: Level: Heart Rate Max: Recovery:

STRENGTH: UPPER BODY & BACK		STRENGTH: LEGS & ABS	
1:	Reps:	1:	Reps:
2:	Reps:	2:	Reps:
3:	Reps:	3:	Reps:
4:	Reps:	4:	Reps:
5:	Reps:	5:	Reps:

FOOD

Breakfast:

Lunch:

Dinner:

Snacks: Crap: Booze:

LIFE

Caring, connecting, committing:

How did you do?   ☐ Amazing   ☐ Not Bad   ☐ Shameful

Plans for tomorrow:

Thursday | | |

How was your night?

Morning mood: Resting Heart Rate:

E X E R C I S E

CARDIO

Time and/or distance: Level: Heart Rate Max: Recovery:

STRENGTH: UPPER BODY & BACK		STRENGTH: LEGS & ABS	
1:	Reps:	1:	Reps:
2:	Reps:	2:	Reps:
3:	Reps:	3:	Reps:
4:	Reps:	4:	Reps:
5:	Reps:	5:	Reps:

F O O D

Breakfast:

Lunch:

Dinner:

Snacks: Crap: Booze:

L I F E

Caring, connecting, committing:

How did you do? ☐ Amazing ☐ Not Bad ☐ Shameful

Plans for tomorrow:

Friday | | |

How was your night?

Morning mood: Resting Heart Rate:

E X E R C I S E

CARDIO

Time and/or distance: Level: Heart Rate Max: Recovery:

STRENGTH: UPPER BODY & BACK		STRENGTH: LEGS & ABS	
1:	Reps:	1:	Reps:
2:	Reps:	2:	Reps:
3:	Reps:	3:	Reps:
4:	Reps:	4:	Reps:
5:	Reps:	5:	Reps:

F O O D

Breakfast:

Lunch:

Dinner:

Snacks: Crap: Booze:

L I F E

Caring, connecting, committing:

How did you do? ☐ Amazing ☐ Not Bad ☐ Shameful

Plans for tomorrow:

Saturday____|__|__|

How was your night?

Morning mood: Resting Heart Rate:

E X E R C I S E

CARDIO

Time and/or distance: Level: Heart Rate Max: Recovery:

STRENGTH: UPPER BODY & BACK		STRENGTH: LEGS & ABS	
1:	Reps:	1:	Reps:
2:	Reps:	2:	Reps:
3:	Reps:	3:	Reps:
4:	Reps:	4:	Reps:
5:	Reps:	5:	Reps:

F O O D

Breakfast:

Lunch:

Dinner:

Snacks: Crap: Booze:

L I F E

Caring, oonncoting, committing:

How did you do? ☐ Amazing ☐ Not Bad ☐ Shameful

Plans for tomorrow:

Sunday____|__|__|

How was your night?

Morning mood: Resting Heart Rate:

E X E R C I S E

CARDIO

Time and/or distance: Level: Heart Rate Max: Recovery:

STRENGTH: UPPER BODY & BACK		STRENGTH: LEGS & ABS	
1:	Reps:	1:	Reps:
2:	Reps:	2:	Reps:
3:	Reps:	3:	Reps:
4:	Reps:	4:	Reps:
5:	Reps:	5:	Reps:

F O O D

Breakfast:

Lunch:

Dinner:

Snacks: Crap: Booze:

L I F E

Caring, connecting, committing:

How did you do? ☐ Amazing ☐ Not Bad ☐ Shameful

Plans for tomorrow:

Exercise & Diet Plan for the Week

	MONDAY	TUESDAY	WEDNESDAY	THURSDAY	FRIDAY	SATURDAY	SUNDAY
CARDIO							
WEIGHTS							

Weight at beginning of week: Weight at end of week:

Goals for the week:

Ideas for caring, connecting, committing:

CHRIS SAYS: **KNOW YOUR "NORMAL" WEIGHT**

Most of us know what we ought to weigh—in other words, not so much what we might actually weigh, but what feels "normal" and right. Know what that set point is for you, and stay there. It's easy to lose the few pounds you just put on if you do it before your body gets used to them . . . and *that* weight becomes the new normal.

Monday ___ | ___ | ___

How was your night?

Morning mood: Resting Heart Rate:

EXERCISE

CARDIO

Time and/or distance: Level: Heart Rate Max: Recovery:

STRENGTH: UPPER BODY & BACK		**STRENGTH: LEGS & ABS**	
1:	Reps:	1:	Reps:
2:	Reps:	2:	Reps:
3:	Reps:	3:	Reps:
4:	Reps:	4:	Reps:
5:	Reps:	5:	Reps:

FOOD

Breakfast:

Lunch:

Dinner:

Snacks: Crap: Booze:

LIFE

Caring, connecting, committing:

How did you do?   ☐ Amazing   ☐ Not Bad   ☐ Shameful

Plans for tomorrow:

Tuesday ___ | |

How was your night?

Morning mood:　　　　　　Resting Heart Rate:

E X E R C I S E

CARDIO

Time and/or distance:　　　　Level:　　　Heart Rate Max:　　　Recovery:

STRENGTH: UPPER BODY & BACK		STRENGTH: LEGS & ABS	
1:	Reps:	1:	Reps:
2:	Reps:	2:	Reps:
3:	Reps:	3:	Reps:
4:	Reps:	4:	Reps:
5:	Reps:	5:	Reps:

F O O D

Breakfast:

Lunch:

Dinner:

Snacks:　　　　　　　　　Crap:　　　　　　Booze:

L I F E

Caring, connecting, committing:

How did you do?　☐Amazing　☐Not Bad　☐Shameful

Plans for tomorrow:

Wednesday ___ | |

How was your night?

Morning mood:　　　　　　Resting Heart Rate:

E X E R C I S E

CARDIO

Time and/or distance:　　　　Level:　　　Heart Rate Max:　　　Recovery:

STRENGTH: UPPER BODY & BACK		STRENGTH: LEGS & ABS	
1:	Reps:	1:	Reps:
2:	Reps:	2:	Reps:
3:	Reps:	3:	Reps:
4:	Reps:	4:	Reps:
5:	Reps:	5:	Reps:

F O O D

Breakfast:

Lunch:

Dinner:

Snacks:　　　　　　　　　Crap:　　　　　　Booze:

L I F E

Caring, connecting, committing:

How did you do?　☐Amazing　☐Not Bad　☐Shameful

Plans for tomorrow:

Thursday ☐ ☐ ☐

How was your night?

Morning mood: Resting Heart Rate:

E X E R C I S E

CARDIO

Time and/or distance: Level: Heart Rate Max: Recovery:

STRENGTH: UPPER BODY & BACK		STRENGTH: LEGS & ABS	
1:	Reps:	1:	Reps:
2:	Reps:	2:	Reps:
3:	Reps:	3:	Reps:
4:	Reps:	4:	Reps:
5:	Reps:	5:	Reps:

F O O D

Breakfast:

Lunch:

Dinner:

Snacks: Crap: Booze:

L I F E

Caring, connecting, committing:

How did you do?   ☐ Amazing   ☐ Not Bad   ☐ Shameful

Plans for tomorrow:

Friday ☐ ☐ ☐

How was your night?

Morning mood: Resting Heart Rate:

E X E R C I S E

CARDIO

Time and/or distance: Level: Heart Rate Max: Recovery:

STRENGTH: UPPER BODY & BACK		STRENGTH: LEGS & ABS	
1:	Reps:	1:	Reps:
2:	Reps:	2:	Reps:
3:	Reps:	3:	Reps:
4:	Reps:	4:	Reps:
5:	Reps:	5:	Reps:

F O O D

Breakfast:

Lunch:

Dinner:

Snacks: Crap: Booze:

L I F E

Caring, connecting, committing:

How did you do?   ☐ Amazing   ☐ Not Bad   ☐ Shameful

Plans for tomorrow:

Saturday____|__|__|

How was your night?	
Morning mood:	Resting Heart Rate:

EXERCISE

CARDIO

Time and/or distance: Level: Heart Rate Max: Recovery:

STRENGTH: UPPER BODY & BACK		STRENGTH: LEGS & ABS	
1:	Reps:	1:	Reps:
2:	Reps:	2:	Reps:
3:	Reps:	3:	Reps:
4:	Reps:	4:	Reps:
5:	Reps:	5:	Reps:

FOOD

Breakfast:

Lunch:

Dinner:

Snacks:	Crap:	Booze:

LIFE

Caring, connecting, committing:

How did you do?   ☐ Amazing   ☐ Not Bad   ☐ Shameful

Plans for tomorrow:

Sunday____|__|__|

How was your night?	
Morning mood:	Resting Heart Rate:

EXERCISE

CARDIO

Time and/or distance: Level: Heart Rate Max: Recovery:

STRENGTH: UPPER BODY & BACK		STRENGTH: LEGS & ABS	
1:	Reps:	1:	Reps:
2:	Reps:	2:	Reps:
3:	Reps:	3:	Reps:
4:	Reps:	4:	Reps:
5:	Reps:	5:	Reps:

FOOD

Breakfast:

Lunch:

Dinner:

Snacks:	Crap:	Booze:

LIFE

Caring, connecting, committing:

How did you do?   ☐ Amazing   ☐ Not Bad   ☐ Shameful

Plans for tomorrow:

35 week
Exercise & Diet Plan for the Week

	MONDAY	TUESDAY	WEDNESDAY	THURSDAY	FRIDAY	SATURDAY	SUNDAY
CARDIO							
WEIGHTS							

Weight at beginning of week: Weight at end of week:

Goals for the week:

Ideas for caring, connecting, committing:

HARRY SAYS: **RUN WITH CARE**

If you're thinking about running, be sure to start very, very slowly. Maybe you can walk for ten minutes, then jog a slow pace for perhaps fifty to one hundred yards, then walk, jog, and so on. Listen to your body! Another option is to add a short walk/run session into your cool-down after your normal gym workout (on the treadmill, the elliptical, or the Stairmaster machine). You'll already be warmed up, so your muscles and tendons have a better shot at tolerating a new exercise.

Monday | | |

How was your night?

Morning mood: Resting Heart Rate:

E X E R C I S E

CARDIO

Time and/or distance: Level: Heart Rate Max: Recovery:

STRENGTH: UPPER BODY & BACK		**STRENGTH: LEGS & ABS**	
1:	Reps:	1:	Reps:
2:	Reps:	2:	Reps:
3:	Reps:	3:	Reps:
4:	Reps:	4:	Reps:
5:	Reps:	5:	Reps:

F O O D

Breakfast:

Lunch:

Dinner:

Snacks: Crap: Booze:

L I F E

Caring, connecting, committing:

How did you do? ☐ Amazing ☐ Not Bad ☐ Shameful

Plans for tomorrow:

Tuesday ___ | | |

How was your night?

Morning mood: Resting Heart Rate:

EXERCISE

CARDIO

Time and/or distance: Level: Heart Rate Max: Recovery:

STRENGTH: UPPER BODY & BACK		STRENGTH: LEGS & ABS	
1:	Reps:	1:	Reps:
2:	Reps:	2:	Reps:
3:	Reps:	3:	Reps:
4:	Reps:	4:	Reps:
5:	Reps:	5:	Reps:

FOOD

Breakfast:

Lunch:

Dinner:

Snacks: Crap: Booze:

LIFE

Caring, connecting, committing:

How did you do?   ☐ Amazing   ☐ Not Bad   ☐ Shameful

Plans for tomorrow:

Wednesday | | |

How was your night?

Morning mood: Resting Heart Rate:

EXERCISE

CARDIO

Time and/or distance: Level: Heart Rate Max: Recovery:

STRENGTH: UPPER BODY & BACK		STRENGTH: LEGS & ABS	
1:	Reps:	1:	Reps:
2:	Reps:	2:	Reps:
3:	Reps:	3:	Reps:
4:	Reps:	4:	Reps:
5:	Reps:	5:	Reps:

FOOD

Breakfast:

Lunch:

Dinner:

Snacks: Crap: Booze:

LIFE

Caring, connecting, committing:

How did you do?   ☐ Amazing   ☐ Not Bad   ☐ Shameful

Plans for tomorrow:

Thursday __|__|__|

How was your night?

Morning mood: Resting Heart Rate:

E X E R C I S E

CARDIO

Time and/or distance: Level: Heart Rate Max: Recovery:

STRENGTH: UPPER BODY & BACK		STRENGTH: LEGS & ABS	
1:	Reps:	1:	Reps:
2:	Reps:	2:	Reps:
3:	Reps:	3:	Reps:
4:	Reps:	4:	Reps:
5:	Reps:	5:	Reps:

F O O D

Breakfast:

Lunch:

Dinner:

Snacks: Crap: Booze:

L I F E

Caring, connecting, committing:

How did you do?   ☐ Amazing ☐ Not Bad ☐ Shameful

Plans for tomorrow:

Friday __|__|__|

How was your night?

Morning mood: Resting Heart Rate:

E X E R C I S E

CARDIO

Time and/or distance: Level: Heart Rate Max: Recovery:

STRENGTH: UPPER BODY & BACK		STRENGTH: LEGS & ABS	
1:	Reps:	1:	Reps:
2:	Reps:	2:	Reps:
3:	Reps:	3:	Reps:
4:	Reps:	4:	Reps:
5:	Reps:	5:	Reps:

F O O D

Breakfast:

Lunch:

Dinner:

Snacks: Crap: Booze:

L I F E

Caring, connecting, committing:

How did you do?   ☐ Amazing ☐ Not Bad ☐ Shameful

Plans for tomorrow:

Saturday _ | | |

How was your night?

Morning mood: Resting Heart Rate:

EXERCISE

CARDIO

| Time and/or distance: | Level: | Heart Rate Max: | Recovery: |

STRENGTH: UPPER BODY & BACK		STRENGTH: LEGS & ABS	
1:	Reps:	1:	Reps:
2:	Reps:	2:	Reps:
3:	Reps:	3:	Reps:
4:	Reps:	4:	Reps:
5:	Reps:	5:	Reps:

FOOD

Breakfast:

Lunch:

Dinner:

| Snacks: | Crap: | Booze: |

LIFE

Caring, connecting, committing.

How did you do?   ☐ Amazing   ☐ Not Bad   ☐ Shameful

Plans for tomorrow:

Sunday _ | | |

How was your night?

Morning mood: Resting Heart Rate:

EXERCISE

CARDIO

| Time and/or distance: | Level: | Heart Rate Max: | Recovery: |

STRENGTH: UPPER BODY & BACK		STRENGTH: LEGS & ABS	
1:	Reps:	1:	Reps:
2:	Reps:	2:	Reps:
3:	Reps:	3:	Reps:
4:	Reps:	4:	Reps:
5:	Reps:	5:	Reps:

FOOD

Breakfast:

Lunch:

Dinner:

| Snacks: | Crap: | Booze: |

LIFE

Caring, connecting, committing:

How did you do?   ☐ Amazing   ☐ Not Bad   ☐ Shameful

Plans for tomorrow:

36 week

Exercise & Diet Plan for the Week

	MONDAY	TUESDAY	WEDNESDAY	THURSDAY	FRIDAY	SATURDAY	SUNDAY
CARDIO							
WEIGHTS							

Weight at beginning of week: _____ Weight at end of week: _____

Goals for the week:

Ideas for caring, connecting, committing:

HARRY SAYS: PLAN YOUR NEXT KEDGE

We hope your first two kedges went well. But no matter what, it's time to step up to the plate and plan another! One year Chris led tough, back-to-back bike trips in Spain and Italy, but that's more than most people can swing. I have a patient who stayed in a tent in the high Sierras and took his grandson hiking ten miles a day. Pick your passion, pick your companions, but *make those plans this week!*

Monday | | |

How was your night?

Morning mood: _____ Resting Heart Rate: _____

E X E R C I S E

CARDIO

Time and/or distance: _____ Level: _____ Heart Rate Max: _____ Recovery: _____

STRENGTH: UPPER BODY & BACK		STRENGTH: LEGS & ABS	
1:	Reps:	1:	Reps:
2:	Reps:	2:	Reps:
3:	Reps:	3:	Reps:
4:	Reps:	4:	Reps:
5:	Reps:	5:	Reps:

F O O D

Breakfast:

Lunch:

Dinner:

Snacks: _____ Crap: _____ Booze: _____

L I F E

Caring, connecting, committing:

How did you do? ☐ Amazing ☐ Not Bad ☐ Shameful

Plans for tomorrow:

Tuesday ⎿_⎿_⎿

How was your night?

Morning mood:　　　　　　Resting Heart Rate:

EXERCISE

CARDIO

Time and/or distance:　　　　Level:　　　Heart Rate Max:　　Recovery:

STRENGTH: UPPER BODY & BACK		STRENGTH: LEGS & ABS	
1:	Reps:	1:	Reps:
2:	Reps:	2:	Reps:
3:	Reps:	3:	Reps:
4:	Reps:	4:	Reps:
5:	Reps:	5:	Reps:

FOOD

Breakfast:

Lunch:

Dinner:

Snacks:　　　　　　　　Crap:　　　　　　Booze:

LIFE

Caring, connecting, committing.

How did you do?　☐ Amazing　☐ Not Bad　☐ Shameful

Plans for tomorrow:

Wednesday ⎿_⎿_⎿

How was your night?

Morning mood:　　　　　　Resting Heart Rate:

EXERCISE

CARDIO

Time and/or distance:　　　　Level:　　　Heart Rate Max:　　Recovery:

STRENGTH: UPPER BODY & BACK		STRENGTH: LEGS & ABS	
1:	Reps:	1:	Reps:
2:	Reps:	2:	Reps:
3:	Reps:	3:	Reps:
4:	Reps:	4:	Reps:
5:	Reps:	5:	Reps:

FOOD

Breakfast:

Lunch:

Dinner:

Snacks:　　　　　　　　Crap:　　　　　　Booze:

LIFE

Caring, connecting, committing:

How did you do?　☐ Amazing　☐ Not Bad　☐ Shameful

Plans for tomorrow:

Thursday ___ | ___ | ___

How was your night?

Morning mood: Resting Heart Rate:

E X E R C I S E

CARDIO

Time and/or distance: Level: Heart Rate Max: Recovery:

STRENGTH: UPPER BODY & BACK		STRENGTH: LEGS & ABS	
1:	Reps:	1:	Reps:
2:	Reps:	2:	Reps:
3:	Reps:	3:	Reps:
4:	Reps:	4:	Reps:
5:	Reps:	5:	Reps:

F O O D

Breakfast:

Lunch:

Dinner:

Snacks: Crap: Booze:

L I F E

Caring, connecting, committing:

How did you do? ☐ Amazing ☐ Not Bad ☐ Shameful

Plans for tomorrow:

Friday ___ | ___ | ___

How was your night?

Morning mood: Resting Heart Rate:

E X E R C I S E

CARDIO

Time and/or distance: Level: Heart Rate Max: Recovery:

STRENGTH: UPPER BODY & BACK		STRENGTH: LEGS & ABS	
1:	Reps:	1:	Reps:
2:	Reps:	2:	Reps:
3:	Reps:	3:	Reps:
4:	Reps:	4:	Reps:
5:	Reps:	5:	Reps:

F O O D

Breakfast:

Lunch:

Dinner:

Snacks: Crap: Booze:

L I F E

Caring, connecting, committing:

How did you do? ☐ Amazing ☐ Not Bad ☐ Shameful

Plans for tomorrow:

Saturday___|___|___

How was your night?

Morning mood: Resting Heart Rate:

EXERCISE

CARDIO

Time and/or distance: Level: Heart Rate Max: Recovery:

STRENGTH: UPPER BODY & BACK		STRENGTH: LEGS & ABS	
1:	Reps:	1:	Reps:
2:	Reps:	2:	Reps:
3:	Reps:	3:	Reps:
4:	Reps:	4:	Reps:
5:	Reps:	5:	Reps:

FOOD

Breakfast:

Lunch:

Dinner:

Snacks: Crap: Booze:

LIFE

Caring, connecting, committing:

How did you do?   ☐ Amazing ☐ Not Bad ☐ Shameful

Plans for tomorrow:

Sunday___|___|___

How was your night?

Morning mood: Resting Heart Rate:

EXERCISE

CARDIO

Time and/or distance: Level: Heart Rate Max: Recovery:

STRENGTH: UPPER BODY & BACK		STRENGTH: LEGS & ABS	
1:	Reps:	1:	Reps:
2:	Reps:	2:	Reps:
3:	Reps:	3:	Reps:
4:	Reps:	4:	Reps:
5:	Reps:	5:	Reps:

FOOD

Breakfast:

Lunch:

Dinner:

Snacks: Crap: Booze:

LIFE

Caring, connecting, committing:

How did you do?   ☐ Amazing ☐ Not Bad ☐ Shameful

Plans for tomorrow:

37 week

Exercise & Diet Plan for the Week

	MONDAY	TUESDAY	WEDNESDAY	THURSDAY	FRIDAY	SATURDAY	SUNDAY
CARDIO							
WEIGHTS							

Weight at beginning of week: _____ Weight at end of week: _____

Goals for the week:

Ideas for caring, connecting, committing:

HARRY SAYS: WHILE YOU'RE AT IT, PLAN ANOTHER KEDGE

Of course, I don't know what time of year you're reading this, but I urge you to plan early for a pre-holiday kedge. Personally, I like to get away for, say, four days of skiing, sometime during the two weeks *before* Christmas or Hanukkah. First, I have my choice of inexpensive destinations. Second, there is something spiritual about ending the year and heading into the holidays on a high note. Plan something hard enough to celebrate your accomplishments and pull you into a new year of youth and fitness. *Whatever you decide to do, plan it this week, because time flies.*

Monday __|__|__

How was your night?

Morning mood: _____ Resting Heart Rate: _____

E X E R C I S E

CARDIO

Time and/or distance: _____ Level: _____ Heart Rate Max: _____ Recovery: _____

STRENGTH: UPPER BODY & BACK		**STRENGTH: LEGS & ABS**	
1:	Reps:	1:	Reps:
2:	Reps:	2:	Reps:
3:	Reps:	3:	Reps:
4:	Reps:	4:	Reps:
5:	Reps:	5:	Reps:

F O O D

Breakfast:

Lunch:

Dinner:

Snacks: _____ Crap: _____ Booze: _____

L I F E

Caring, connecting, committing:

How did you do? ☐ Amazing ☐ Not Bad ☐ Shameful

Plans for tomorrow:

Tuesday_____ | | |

How was your night?

Morning mood: Resting Heart Rate:

E X E R C I S E

CARDIO

Time and/or distance: Level: Heart Rate Max: Recovery:

STRENGTH: UPPER BODY & BACK		STRENGTH: LEGS & ABS	
1:	Reps:	1:	Reps:
2:	Reps:	2:	Reps:
3:	Reps:	3:	Reps:
4:	Reps:	4:	Reps:
5:	Reps:	5:	Reps:

F O O D

Breakfast:

Lunch:

Dinner:

Snacks: Crap: Booze:

L I F E

Caring, connecting, committing:

How did you do?   ☐ Amazing   ☐ Not Bad   ☐ Shameful

Plans for tomorrow:

Wednesday_____ | | |

How was your night?

Morning mood: Resting Heart Rate:

E X E R C I S E

CARDIO

Time and/or distance: Level: Heart Rate Max: Recovery:

STRENGTH: UPPER BODY & BACK		STRENGTH: LEGS & ABS	
1:	Reps:	1:	Reps:
2:	Reps:	2:	Reps:
3:	Reps:	3:	Reps:
4:	Reps:	4:	Reps:
5:	Reps:	5:	Reps:

F O O D

Breakfast:

Lunch:

Dinner:

Snacks: Crap: Booze:

L I F E

Caring, connecting, committing:

How did you do?   ☐ Amazing   ☐ Not Bad   ☐ Shameful

Plans for tomorrow:

Thursday ___ | ___ | ___ |

How was your night?

Morning mood: Resting Heart Rate:

E X E R C I S E

CARDIO

Time and/or distance: Level: Heart Rate Max: Recovery:

STRENGTH: UPPER BODY & BACK		**STRENGTH: LEGS & ABS**	
1:	Reps:	1:	Reps:
2:	Reps:	2:	Reps:
3:	Reps:	3:	Reps:
4:	Reps:	4:	Reps:
5:	Reps:	5:	Reps:

F O O D

Breakfast:

Lunch:

Dinner:

Snacks: Crap: Booze:

L I F E

Caring, connecting, committing:

How did you do?   ☐ Amazing   ☐ Not Bad   ☐ Shameful

Plans for tomorrow:

Friday ___ | ___ | ___ |

How was your night?

Morning mood: Resting Heart Rate:

E X E R C I S E

CARDIO

Time and/or distance: Level: Heart Rate Max: Recovery:

STRENGTH: UPPER BODY & BACK		**STRENGTH: LEGS & ABS**	
1:	Reps:	1:	Reps:
2:	Reps:	2:	Reps:
3:	Reps:	3:	Reps:
4:	Reps:	4:	Reps:
5:	Reps:	5:	Reps:

F O O D

Breakfast:

Lunch:

Dinner:

Snacks: Crap: Booze:

L I F E

Caring, connecting, committing:

How did you do?   ☐ Amazing   ☐ Not Bad   ☐ Shameful

Plans for tomorrow:

Saturday ___ | | |

How was your night?

Morning mood: Resting Heart Rate:

EXERCISE

CARDIO

Time and/or distance: Level: Heart Rate Max: Recovery:

STRENGTH: UPPER BODY & BACK		STRENGTH: LEGS & ABS	
1:	Reps:	1:	Reps:
2:	Reps:	2:	Reps:
3:	Reps:	3:	Reps:
4:	Reps:	4:	Reps:
5:	Reps:	5:	Reps:

FOOD

Breakfast:

Lunch:

Dinner:

Snacks: Crap: Booze:

LIFE

Caring, connecting, committing:

How did you do?   ☐ Amazing   ☐ Not Bad   ☐ Shameful

Plans for tomorrow:

Sunday ___ | | |

How was your night?

Morning mood: Resting Heart Rate:

EXERCISE

CARDIO

Time and/or distance: Level: Heart Rate Max: Recovery:

STRENGTH: UPPER BODY & BACK		STRENGTH: LEGS & ABS	
1:	Reps:	1:	Reps:
2:	Reps:	2:	Reps:
3:	Reps:	3:	Reps:
4:	Reps:	4:	Reps:
5:	Reps:	5:	Reps:

FOOD

Breakfast:

Lunch:

Dinner:

Snacks: Crap: Booze:

LIFE

Caring, connecting, committing:

How did you do?   ☐ Amazing   ☐ Not Bad   ☐ Shameful

Plans for tomorrow:

Exercise & Diet Plan for the Week

	MONDAY	TUESDAY	WEDNESDAY	THURSDAY	FRIDAY	SATURDAY	SUNDAY
CARDIO							
WEIGHTS							

Weight at beginning of week: Weight at end of week:

Goals for the week:

Ideas for caring, connecting, committing:

HARRY SAYS: TAKE CARE OF YOUR KNEES

If you're suffering from knee pain—as a lot of people are—ask your doctor if you can try strength training. If you can, remember that the key is consistent, very slow progression. (You need to listen to your joints, not your muscles, which will get stronger faster.) Move slowly, watch your form, and use light weights. You are going to end up stronger than the people tossing too much weight around . . . and you'll have much better joints!

Monday | | |

How was your night?

Morning mood: Resting Heart Rate:

EXERCISE

CARDIO

Time and/or distance: Level: Heart Rate Max: Recovery:

STRENGTH: UPPER BODY & BACK		STRENGTH: LEGS & ABS	
1:	Reps:	1:	Reps:
2:	Reps:	2:	Reps:
3:	Reps:	3:	Reps:
4:	Reps:	4:	Reps:
5:	Reps:	5:	Reps:

FOOD

Breakfast:

Lunch:

Dinner:

Snacks: Crap: Booze:

LIFE

Caring, connecting, committing:

How did you do? ☐ Amazing ☐ Not Bad ☐ Shameful

Plans for tomorrow:

Tuesday ☐ ☐ ☐

How was your night?

Morning mood: Resting Heart Rate:

EXERCISE

CARDIO

Time and/or distance: Level: Heart Rate Max: Recovery:

STRENGTH: UPPER BODY & BACK		STRENGTH: LEGS & ABS	
1:	Reps:	1:	Reps:
2:	Reps:	2:	Reps:
3:	Reps:	3:	Reps:
4:	Reps:	4:	Reps:
5:	Reps:	5:	Reps:

FOOD

Breakfast:

Lunch:

Dinner:

Snacks: Crap: Booze:

LIFE

Caring, connecting, committing:

How did you do?   ☐ Amazing ☐ Not Bad ☐ Shameful

Plans for tomorrow:

Wednesday ☐ ☐ ☐

How was your night?

Morning mood: Resting Heart Rate:

EXERCISE

CARDIO

Time and/or distance: Level: Heart Rate Max: Recovery:

STRENGTH: UPPER BODY & BACK		STRENGTH: LEGS & ABS	
1:	Reps:	1:	Reps:
2:	Reps:	2:	Reps:
3:	Reps:	3:	Reps:
4:	Reps:	4:	Reps:
5:	Reps:	5:	Reps:

FOOD

Breakfast:

Lunch:

Dinner:

Snacks: Crap: Booze:

LIFE

Caring, connecting, committing:

How did you do?   ☐ Amazing ☐ Not Bad ☐ Shameful

Plans for tomorrow:

Thursday _ | | _

How was your night?

Morning mood: Resting Heart Rate:

E X E R C I S E

CARDIO

Time and/or distance: Level: Heart Rate Max: Recovery:

STRENGTH: UPPER BODY & BACK		**STRENGTH: LEGS & ABS**	
1:	Reps:	1:	Reps:
2:	Reps:	2:	Reps:
3:	Reps:	3:	Reps:
4:	Reps:	4:	Reps:
5:	Reps:	5:	Reps:

F O O D

Breakfast:

Lunch:

Dinner:

Snacks: Crap: Booze:

L I F E

Caring, connecting, committing:

How did you do?   ☐ Amazing   ☐ Not Bad   ☐ Shameful

Plans for tomorrow:

Friday _ | | _

How was your night?

Morning mood: Resting Heart Rate:

E X E R C I S E

CARDIO

Time and/or distance: Level: Heart Rate Max: Recovery:

STRENGTH: UPPER BODY & BACK		**STRENGTH: LEGS & ABS**	
1:	Reps:	1:	Reps:
2:	Reps:	2:	Reps:
3:	Reps:	3:	Reps:
4:	Reps:	4:	Reps:
5:	Reps:	5:	Reps:

F O O D

Breakfast:

Lunch:

Dinner:

Snacks: Crap: Booze:

L I F E

Caring, connecting, committing:

How did you do?   ☐ Amazing   ☐ Not Bad   ☐ Shameful

Plans for tomorrow:

Saturday___|__|__|

How was your night?

Morning mood: Resting Heart Rate:

EXERCISE

CARDIO

Time and/or distance: Level: Heart Rate Max: Recovery:

STRENGTH: UPPER BODY & BACK		STRENGTH: LEGS & ABS	
1:	Reps:	1:	Reps:
2:	Reps:	2:	Reps:
3:	Reps:	3:	Reps:
4:	Reps:	4:	Reps:
5:	Reps:	5:	Reps:

FOOD

Breakfast:

Lunch:

Dinner:

Snacks: Crap: Booze:

LIFE

Caring, connecting, committing:

How did you do?   ☐ Amazing   ☐ Not Bad   ☐ Shameful

Plans for tomorrow:

Sunday___|__|__|

How was your night?

Morning mood: Resting Heart Rate:

EXERCISE

CARDIO

Time and/or distance: Level: Heart Rate Max: Recovery:

STRENGTH: UPPER BODY & BACK		STRENGTH: LEGS & ABS	
1:	Reps:	1:	Reps:
2:	Reps:	2:	Reps:
3:	Reps:	3:	Reps:
4:	Reps.	4.	Reps:
5.	Reps:	5:	Reps:

FOOD

Breakfast:

Lunch:

Dinner:

Snacks: Crap: Booze:

LIFE

Caring, connecting, committing:

How did you do?   ☐ Amazing   ☐ Not Bad   ☐ Shameful

Plans for tomorrow:

39 week Exercise & Diet Plan for the Week

	MONDAY	TUESDAY	WEDNESDAY	THURSDAY	FRIDAY	SATURDAY	SUNDAY
CARDIO							
WEIGHTS							

Weight at beginning of week: Weight at end of week:

Goals for the week:

Ideas for caring, connecting, committing:

HARRY SAYS: **TAKE A CUE FROM YOGA**

Holding a stretch for around thirty seconds is much more beneficial than any of the calisthenics-type stretching we all learned in high school. And doing it *after* a workout, when your muscles are warmer, looser, and more flexible is the only thing that makes sense to me. However, plenty of people, especially runners, swear that stretching before exercise limbers them up. Bottom line: Listen carefully to your own body.

Monday | | |

How was your night?

Morning mood: Resting Heart Rate:

EXERCISE

CARDIO

Time and/or distance: Level: Heart Rate Max: Recovery:

STRENGTH: UPPER BODY & BACK		STRENGTH: LEGS & ABS	
1:	Reps:	1:	Reps:
2:	Reps:	2:	Reps:
3:	Reps:	3:	Reps:
4:	Reps:	4:	Reps:
5:	Reps:	5:	Reps:

FOOD

Breakfast:

Lunch:

Dinner:

Snacks: Crap: Booze:

LIFE

Caring, connecting, committing:

How did you do?   ☐ Amazing   ☐ Not Bad   ☐ Shameful

Plans for tomorrow:

Tuesday ___ | ___ | ___

How was your night?

Morning mood: ___ Resting Heart Rate: ___

E X E R C I S E

CARDIO

Time and/or distance: ___ Level: ___ Heart Rate Max: ___ Recovery: ___

STRENGTH: UPPER BODY & BACK		STRENGTH: LEGS & ABS	
1:	Reps:	1:	Reps:
2:	Reps:	2:	Reps:
3:	Reps:	3:	Reps:
4:	Reps:	4:	Reps:
5:	Reps:	5:	Reps:

F O O D

Breakfast:

Lunch:

Dinner:

Snacks: ___ Crap: ___ Booze: ___

L I F E

Caring, connecting, committing.

How did you do? ☐ Amazing ☐ Not Bad ☐ Shameful

Plans for tomorrow:

Wednesday ___ | ___ | ___

How was your night?

Morning mood: ___ Resting Heart Rate: ___

E X E R C I S E

CARDIO

Time and/or distance: ___ Level: ___ Heart Rate Max: ___ Recovery: ___

STRENGTH: UPPER BODY & BACK		STRENGTH: LEGS & ABS	
1:	Reps:	1:	Reps:
2:	Reps:	2:	Reps:
3:	Reps:	3:	Reps:
4:	Reps:	4:	Reps:
5:	Reps:	5:	Reps:

F O O D

Breakfast:

Lunch:

Dinner:

Snacks: ___ Crap: ___ Booze: ___

L I F E

Caring, connecting, committing:

How did you do? ☐ Amazing ☐ Not Bad ☐ Shameful

Plans for tomorrow:

Thursday ____|___|___

How was your night?

Morning mood: Resting Heart Rate:

EXERCISE

CARDIO

Time and/or distance: Level: Heart Rate Max: Recovery:

STRENGTH: UPPER BODY & BACK		STRENGTH: LEGS & ABS	
1:	Reps:	1:	Reps:
2:	Reps:	2:	Reps:
3:	Reps:	3:	Reps:
4:	Reps:	4:	Reps:
5:	Reps:	5:	Reps:

FOOD

Breakfast:

Lunch:

Dinner:

Snacks: Crap: Booze:

LIFE

Caring, connecting, committing:

How did you do?   ☐ Amazing   ☐ Not Bad   ☐ Shameful

Plans for tomorrow:

Friday ____|___|___

How was your night?

Morning mood: Resting Heart Rate:

EXERCISE

CARDIO

Time and/or distance: Level: Heart Rate Max: Recovery:

STRENGTH: UPPER BODY & BACK		STRENGTH: LEGS & ABS	
1:	Reps:	1:	Reps:
2:	Reps:	2:	Reps:
3:	Reps:	3:	Reps:
4:	Reps:	4:	Reps:
5:	Reps:	5:	Reps:

FOOD

Breakfast:

Lunch:

Dinner:

Snacks: Crap: Booze:

LIFE

Caring, connecting, committing:

How did you do?   ☐ Amazing   ☐ Not Bad   ☐ Shameful

Plans for tomorrow:

Saturday␣␣␣

How was your night?

Morning mood:　　　　Resting Heart Rate:

E X E R C I S E

CARDIO

Time and/or distance:　　　Level:　　　Heart Rate Max:　　　Recovery:

STRENGTH: UPPER BODY & BACK		STRENGTH: LEGS & ABS	
1:	Reps:	1:	Reps:
2:	Reps:	2:	Reps:
3:	Reps:	3:	Reps:
4:	Reps:	4:	Reps:
5:	Reps:	5:	Reps:

F O O D

Breakfast:

Lunch:

Dinner:

Snacks:　　　　　Crap:　　　　　Booze:

L I F E

Caring, connecting, committing:

How did you do?　☐ Amazing　☐ Not Bad　☐ Shameful

Plans for tomorrow:

Sunday␣␣␣

How was your night?

Morning mood:　　　　Resting Heart Rate:

E X E R C I S E

CARDIO

Time and/or distance:　　　Level:　　　Heart Rate Max:　　　Recovery:

STRENGTH: UPPER BODY & BACK		STRENGTH: LEGS & ABS	
1:	Reps:	1:	Reps:
2:	Reps:	2:	Reps:
3:	Reps:	3:	Reps:
4:	Reps:	4:	Reps:
5:	Reps:	5:	Reps:

F O O D

Breakfast:

Lunch:

Dinner:

Snacks:　　　　　Crap:　　　　　Booze:

L I F E

Caring, connecting, committing:

How did you do?　☐ Amazing　☐ Not Bad　☐ Shameful

Plans for tomorrow:

40
week

Exercise & Diet Plan for the Week

	MONDAY	TUESDAY	WEDNESDAY	THURSDAY	FRIDAY	SATURDAY	SUNDAY
CARDIO							
WEIGHTS							

Weight at beginning of week: _____ Weight at end of week: _____

Goals for the week: _____

Ideas for caring, connecting, committing: _____

HARRY SAYS: **KEEP GOING IF YOU DON'T LOSE WEIGHT**

If you're trying to lose weight, you need to be patient, since you shouldn't lose more than half a pound a week. But if you find yourself not losing weight, or even if you have a week when you gain weight, don't stop exercising! Getting fit and managing weight are completely separate goals—related, to be sure, but essentially separate.

Monday ⎵⎵⎵

How was your night? _____

Morning mood: _____ Resting Heart Rate: _____

E X E R C I S E

CARDIO

Time and/or distance: _____ Level: _____ Heart Rate Max: _____ Recovery: _____

STRENGTH: UPPER BODY & BACK		**STRENGTH: LEGS & ABS**	
1:	Reps:	1:	Reps:
2:	Reps:	2:	Reps:
3:	Reps:	3:	Reps:
4:	Reps:	4:	Reps:
5:	Reps:	5:	Reps:

F O O D

Breakfast:

Lunch:

Dinner:

Snacks: _____ Crap: _____ Booze: _____

L I F E

Caring, connecting, committing:

How did you do? ☐ Amazing ☐ Not Bad ☐ Shameful

Plans for tomorrow:

Tuesday __ | __ | __

How was your night?

Morning mood: Resting Heart Rate:

E X E R C I S E

CARDIO

Time and/or distance: Level: Heart Rate Max: Recovery:

STRENGTH: UPPER BODY & BACK		STRENGTH: LEGS & ABS	
1:	Reps:	1:	Reps:
2:	Reps:	2:	Reps:
3:	Reps:	3:	Reps:
4:	Reps:	4:	Reps:
5:	Reps:	5:	Reps:

F O O D

Breakfast:

Lunch:

Dinner:

Snacks: Crap: Booze:

L I F E

Caring, connecting, committing:

How did you do? ☐ Amazing ☐ Not Bad ☐ Shameful

Plans for tomorrow:

Wednesday __ | __ | __

How was your night?

Morning mood: Resting Heart Rate:

E X E R C I S E

CARDIO

Time and/or distance: Level: Heart Rate Max: Recovery:

STRENGTH: UPPER BODY & BACK		STRENGTH: LEGS & ABS	
1:	Reps:	1:	Reps:
2:	Reps:	2:	Reps:
3:	Reps:	3:	Reps:
4:	Reps:	4:	Reps:
5:	Reps:	5:	Reps:

F O O D

Breakfast:

Lunch:

Dinner:

Snacks: Crap: Booze:

L I F E

Caring, connecting, committing:

How did you do? ☐ Amazing ☐ Not Bad ☐ Shameful

Plans for tomorrow:

Thursday ___ | | |

How was your night?

Morning mood: Resting Heart Rate:

E X E R C I S E

CARDIO

Time and/or distance: Level: Heart Rate Max: Recovery:

STRENGTH: UPPER BODY & BACK		STRENGTH: LEGS & ABS	
1:	Reps:	1:	Reps:
2:	Reps:	2:	Reps:
3:	Reps:	3:	Reps:
4:	Reps:	4:	Reps:
5:	Reps:	5:	Reps:

F O O D

Breakfast:

Lunch:

Dinner:

Snacks: Crap: Booze:

L I F E

Caring, connecting, committing:

How did you do? ☐ Amazing ☐ Not Bad ☐ Shameful

Plans for tomorrow:

Friday ___ | | |

How was your night?

Morning mood: Resting Heart Rate:

E X E R C I S E

CARDIO

Time and/or distance: Level: Heart Rate Max: Recovery:

STRENGTH: UPPER BODY & BACK		STRENGTH: LEGS & ABS	
1:	Reps:	1:	Reps:
2:	Reps:	2:	Reps:
3:	Reps:	3:	Reps:
4:	Reps:	4:	Reps:
5:	Reps:	5:	Reps:

F O O D

Breakfast:

Lunch:

Dinner:

Snacks: Crap: Booze:

L I F E

Caring, connecting, committing:

How did you do? ☐ Amazing ☐ Not Bad ☐ Shameful

Plans for tomorrow:

Saturday___|___|___

How was your night?

Morning mood: Resting Heart Rate:

E X E R C I S E

CARDIO

Time and/or distance: Level: Heart Rate Max: Recovery:

STRENGTH: UPPER BODY & BACK		STRENGTH: LEGS & ABS	
1:	Reps:	1:	Reps:
2:	Reps:	2:	Reps:
3:	Reps:	3:	Reps:
4:	Reps:	4:	Reps:
5:	Reps:	5:	Reps:

F O O D

Breakfast:

Lunch:

Dinner:

Snacks: Crap: Booze:

L I F E

Caring, connecting, committing:

How did you do?   ☐ Amazing   ☐ Not Bad   ☐ Shameful

Plans for tomorrow:

Sunday___|___|___

How was your night?

Morning mood: Resting Heart Rate:

E X E R C I S E

CARDIO

Time and/or distance: Level: Heart Rate Max: Recovery:

STRENGTH: UPPER BODY & BACK		STRENGTH: LEGS & ABS	
1:	Reps:	1:	Reps:
2:	Reps:	2:	Reps:
3:	Reps:	3:	Reps:
4:	Reps:	4:	Reps:
5:	Reps:	5:	Reps:

F O O D

Breakfast:

Lunch:

Dinner:

Snacks: Crap: Booze:

L I F E

Caring, connecting, committing:

How did you do?   ☐ Amazing   ☐ Not Bad   ☐ Shameful

Plans for tomorrow:

Exercise & Diet Plan for the Week

	MONDAY	TUESDAY	WEDNESDAY	THURSDAY	FRIDAY	SATURDAY	SUNDAY
CARDIO							
WEIGHTS							

Weight at beginning of week: _____ Weight at end of week: _____

Goals for the week: _____

Ideas for caring, connecting, committing: _____

HARRY SAYS: **MAKE EXERCISE SOCIAL**

Working out with your friends can be fun. Not necessarily barrel-of-laughs fun, but interesting fun, particularly if it's followed by coffee, a drink, a movie, or anything else you want. All you need to do is structure it so everyone *ends* at the same time, even if they start at different times. Take the lead in this. Be the organizer even—perhaps especially—if it's not your native temperament. That way you are making the biggest commitment and you are most likely to keep showing up.

Monday | | |

How was your night? _____

Morning mood: _____ Resting Heart Rate: _____

E X E R C I S E

CARDIO

Time and/or distance: _____ Level: _____ Heart Rate Max: _____ Recovery: _____

STRENGTH: UPPER BODY & BACK		STRENGTH: LEGS & ABS	
1:	Reps:	1:	Reps:
2:	Reps:	2:	Reps:
3:	Reps:	3:	Reps:
4:	Reps:	4:	Reps:
5:	Reps:	5:	Reps:

F O O D

Breakfast:

Lunch:

Dinner:

Snacks: _____ Crap: _____ Booze: _____

L I F E

Caring, connecting, committing:

How did you do? ☐ Amazing ☐ Not Bad ☐ Shameful

Plans for tomorrow:

Tuesday _____

How was your night?

Morning mood: _____ Resting Heart Rate:

EXERCISE

CARDIO

Time and/or distance: ____ Level: ____ Heart Rate Max: ____ Recovery:

STRENGTH: UPPER BODY & BACK		STRENGTH: LEGS & ABS	
1:	Reps:	1:	Reps:
2:	Reps:	2:	Reps:
3:	Reps:	3:	Reps:
4:	Reps:	4:	Reps:
5:	Reps:	5:	Reps:

FOOD

Breakfast:

Lunch:

Dinner:

Snacks: ____ Crap: ____ Booze:

LIFE

Caring, connecting, committing:

How did you do? ☐ Amazing ☐ Not Bad ☐ Shameful

Plans for tomorrow:

Wednesday _____

How was your night?

Morning mood: _____ Resting Heart Rate:

EXERCISE

CARDIO

Time and/or distance: ____ Level: ____ Heart Rate Max: ____ Recovery:

STRENGTH: UPPER BODY & BACK		STRENGTH: LEGS & ABS	
1:	Reps:	1:	Reps:
2:	Reps:	2:	Reps:
3:	Reps:	3:	Reps:
4:	Reps:	4:	Reps:
5:	Reps:	5:	Reps:

FOOD

Breakfast:

Lunch:

Dinner:

Snacks: ____ Crap: ____ Booze:

LIFE

Caring, connecting, committing:

How did you do? ☐ Amazing ☐ Not Bad ☐ Shameful

Plans for tomorrow:

Thursday ⎵ | |

How was your night?

Morning mood: Resting Heart Rate:

E X E R C I S E

CARDIO

Time and/or distance: Level: Heart Rate Max: Recovery:

STRENGTH: UPPER BODY & BACK		STRENGTH: LEGS & ABS	
1:	Reps:	1:	Reps:
2:	Reps:	2:	Reps:
3:	Reps:	3:	Reps:
4:	Reps:	4:	Reps:
5:	Reps:	5:	Reps:

F O O D

Breakfast:

Lunch:

Dinner:

Snacks: Crap: Booze:

L I F E

Caring, connecting, committing:

How did you do?   ☐ Amazing ☐ Not Bad ☐ Shameful

Plans for tomorrow:

Friday ⎵ | |

How was your night?

Morning mood: Resting Heart Rate:

E X E R C I S E

CARDIO

Time and/or distance: Level: Heart Rate Max: Recovery:

STRENGTH: UPPER BODY & BACK		STRENGTH: LEGS & ABS	
1:	Reps:	1:	Reps:
2:	Reps:	2:	Reps:
3:	Reps:	3:	Reps:
4:	Reps:	4:	Reps:
5:	Reps:	5:	Reps:

F O O D

Breakfast:

Lunch:

Dinner:

Snacks: Crap: Booze:

L I F E

Caring, connecting, committing:

How did you do?   ☐ Amazing ☐ Not Bad ☐ Shameful

Plans for tomorrow:

Saturday ___ | | |

How was your night?

Morning mood: Resting Heart Rate:

E X E R C I S E

CARDIO

Time and/or distance: Level: Heart Rate Max: Recovery:

STRENGTH: UPPER BODY & BACK		**STRENGTH: LEGS & ABS**	
1:	Reps:	1:	Reps:
2:	Reps:	2:	Reps:
3:	Reps:	3:	Reps:
4:	Reps:	4:	Reps:
5:	Reps:	5:	Reps:

F O O D

Breakfast:

Lunch:

Dinner:

Snacks: Crap: Booze:

L I F E

Caring, connecting, committing:

How did you do?   ☐ Amazing ☐ Not Bad ☐ Shameful

Plans for tomorrow:

Sunday ___ | | |

How was your night?

Morning mood: Resting Heart Rate:

E X E R C I S E

CARDIO

Time and/or distance: Level: Heart Rate Max: Recovery:

STRENGTH: UPPER BODY & BACK		**STRENGTH: LEGS & ABS**	
1:	Reps:	1:	Reps:
2:	Reps:	2:	Reps:
3:	Reps:	3:	Reps:
4:	Reps:	4:	Reps:
5:	Reps:	5:	Reps:

F O O D

Breakfast:

Lunch:

Dinner:

Snacks: Crap: Booze:

L I F E

Caring, connecting, committing:

How did you do?   ☐ Amazing ☐ Not Bad ☐ Shameful

Plans for tomorrow:

42 week — Exercise & Diet Plan for the Week

	MONDAY	TUESDAY	WEDNESDAY	THURSDAY	FRIDAY	SATURDAY	SUNDAY
CARDIO							
WEIGHTS							

Weight at beginning of week: Weight at end of week:

Goals for the week:

Ideas for caring, connecting, committing:

CHRIS SAYS: NEVER USE AGE AS AN EXCUSE

It is never too late to begin this stuff. If you're somewhere between forty and sixty, fine. But if you (or your parents or grandparents) are in your seventies, eighties, or even nineties, don't think you can't reap huge benefits from exercising. You can. And you must.

Monday ⎵⎵⎵

How was your night?

Morning mood: Resting Heart Rate:

EXERCISE

CARDIO

Time and/or distance: Level: Heart Rate Max: Recovery:

STRENGTH: UPPER BODY & BACK		STRENGTH: LEGS & ABS	
1:	Reps:	1:	Reps:
2:	Reps:	2:	Reps:
3:	Reps:	3:	Reps:
4:	Reps:	4:	Reps:
5:	Reps:	5:	Reps:

FOOD

Breakfast:

Lunch:

Dinner:

Snacks: Crap: Booze:

LIFE

Caring, connecting, committing:

How did you do?   ☐ Amazing   ☐ Not Bad   ☐ Shameful

Plans for tomorrow:

Tuesday___|___|___|

How was your night?

Morning mood: Resting Heart Rate:

EXERCISE

CARDIO

Time and/or distance: Level: Heart Rate Max: Recovery:

STRENGTH: UPPER BODY & BACK		STRENGTH: LEGS & ABS	
1:	Reps:	1:	Reps:
2:	Reps:	2:	Reps:
3:	Reps:	3:	Reps:
4:	Reps:	4:	Reps:
5:	Reps:	5:	Reps:

FOOD

Breakfast:

Lunch:

Dinner:

Snacks: Crap: Booze:

LIFE

Caring, connecting, committing:

How did you do? ☐ Amazing ☐ Not Bad ☐ Shameful

Plans for tomorrow:

Wednesday___|___|___|

How was your night?

Morning mood: Resting Heart Rate:

EXERCISE

CARDIO

Time and/or distance: Level: Heart Rate Max: Recovery:

STRENGTH: UPPER BODY & BACK		STRENGTH: LEGS & ABS	
1:	Reps:	1:	Reps:
2:	Reps:	2:	Reps:
3:	Reps:	3:	Reps:
4:	Reps:	4:	Reps:
5:	Reps:	5:	Reps:

FOOD

Breakfast:

Lunch:

Dinner:

Snacks: Crap: Booze:

LIFE

Caring, connecting, committing:

How did you do? ☐ Amazing ☐ Not Bad ☐ Shameful

Plans for tomorrow:

Thursday_ | _ | _ |

How was your night?

Morning mood: Resting Heart Rate:

E X E R C I S E

CARDIO

Time and/or distance: Level: Heart Rate Max: Recovery:

STRENGTH: UPPER BODY & BACK		**STRENGTH: LEGS & ABS**	
1:	Reps:	1:	Reps:
2:	Reps:	2:	Reps:
3:	Reps:	3:	Reps:
4:	Reps:	4:	Reps:
5:	Reps:	5:	Reps:

F O O D

Breakfast:

Lunch:

Dinner:

Snacks: Crap: Booze:

L I F E

Caring, connecting, committing:

How did you do?   ☐ Amazing   ☐ Not Bad   ☐ Shameful

Plans for tomorrow:

Friday_ | _ | _ |

How was your night?

Morning mood: Resting Heart Rate:

E X E R C I S E

CARDIO

Time and/or distance: Level: Heart Rate Max: Recovery:

STRENGTH: UPPER BODY & BACK		**STRENGTH: LEGS & ABS**	
1:	Reps:	1:	Reps:
2:	Reps:	2:	Reps:
3:	Reps:	3:	Reps:
4:	Reps:	4:	Reps:
5:	Reps:	5:	Reps:

F O O D

Breakfast:

Lunch:

Dinner:

Snacks: Crap: Booze:

L I F E

Caring, connecting, committing:

How did you do?   ☐ Amazing   ☐ Not Bad   ☐ Shameful

Plans for tomorrow:

Saturday___|___|___

How was your night?	
Morning mood:	Resting Heart Rate:

E X E R C I S E

CARDIO

Time and/or distance: Level: Heart Rate Max: Recovery:

STRENGTH: UPPER BODY & BACK		STRENGTH: LEGS & ABS	
1:	Reps:	1:	Reps:
2:	Reps:	2:	Reps:
3:	Reps:	3:	Reps:
4:	Reps:	4:	Reps:
5:	Reps:	5:	Reps:

F O O D

Breakfast:

Lunch:

Dinner:

Snacks: Crap: Booze:

L I F E

Caring, connecting, committing:

How did you do?   ☐ Amazing ☐ Not Bad ☐ Shameful

Plans for tomorrow:

Sunday___|___|___

How was your night?	
Morning mood:	Resting Heart Rate:

E X E R C I S E

CARDIO

Time and/or distance: Level: Heart Rate Max: Recovery:

STRENGTH: UPPER BODY & BACK		STRENGTH: LEGS & ABS	
1:	Reps:	1:	Reps:
2:	Reps:	2:	Reps:
3:	Reps:	3:	Reps:
4:	Reps:	4:	Reps:
5:	Reps:	5:	Reps:

F O O D

Breakfast:

Lunch:

Dinner:

Snacks: Crap: Booze:

L I F E

Caring, connecting, committing:

How did you do?   ☐ Amazing ☐ Not Bad ☐ Shameful

Plans for tomorrow:

43 week

Exercise & Diet Plan for the Week

	MONDAY	TUESDAY	WEDNESDAY	THURSDAY	FRIDAY	SATURDAY	SUNDAY
CARDIO							
WEIGHTS							

Weight at beginning of week: Weight at end of week:

Goals for the week:

Ideas for caring, connecting, committing:

HARRY SAYS: GET RID OF JET LAG

Here's some advice for you travelers: Work out long and hard the day you're flying (or the day before). Drink a lot of water. If you have time in the airport, move or stretch. Continue to hydrate and avoid alcohol. When you arrive at your destination, get some light exercise. The next morning, get up on local time, no matter how much sleep you've had. Get in some more light exercise. Twenty minutes is usually enough. Drink lots of water. End of sermon.

Monday ___|___|___|

How was your night?

Morning mood: Resting Heart Rate:

E X E R C I S E

CARDIO

Time and/or distance: Level: Heart Rate Max: Recovery:

STRENGTH: UPPER BODY & BACK		STRENGTH: LEGS & ABS	
1:	Reps:	1:	Reps:
2:	Reps:	2:	Reps:
3:	Reps:	3:	Reps:
4:	Reps:	4:	Reps:
5:	Reps:	5:	Reps:

F O O D

Breakfast:

Lunch:

Dinner:

Snacks: Crap: Booze:

L I F E

Caring, connecting, committing:

How did you do? ☐ Amazing ☐ Not Bad ☐ Shameful

Plans for tomorrow:

Tuesday _ | | |

How was your night?

Morning mood: Resting Heart Rate:

E X E R C I S E

CARDIO

Time and/or distance: Level: Heart Rate Max: Recovery:

STRENGTH: UPPER BODY & BACK		**STRENGTH: LEGS & ABS**	
1:	Reps:	1:	Reps:
2:	Reps:	2:	Reps:
3:	Reps:	3:	Reps:
4:	Reps:	4:	Reps:
5:	Reps:	5:	Reps:

F O O D

Breakfast:

Lunch:

Dinner:

Snacks: Crap: Booze:

L I F E

Caring, connecting, committing:

How did you do?   ☐ Amazing ☐ Not Bad ☐ Shameful

Plans for tomorrow:

Wednesday _ | | |

How was your night?

Morning mood: Resting Heart Rate:

E X E R C I S E

CARDIO

Time and/or distance: Level: Heart Rate Max: Recovery:

STRENGTH: UPPER BODY & BACK		**STRENGTH: LEGS & ABS**	
1:	Reps:	1:	Reps:
2:	Reps:	2:	Reps:
3:	Reps:	3:	Reps:
4:	Reps:	4:	Reps:
5:	Reps:	5:	Reps:

F O O D

Breakfast:

Lunch:

Dinner:

Snacks: Crap: Booze:

L I F E

Caring, connecting, committing:

How did you do?   ☐ Amazing ☐ Not Bad ☐ Shameful

Plans for tomorrow:

Thursday ☐ ☐ ☐

How was your night?

Morning mood: Resting Heart Rate:

EXERCISE

CARDIO

Time and/or distance: Level: Heart Rate Max: Recovery:

STRENGTH: UPPER BODY & BACK		STRENGTH: LEGS & ABS	
1:	Reps:	1:	Reps:
2:	Reps:	2:	Reps:
3:	Reps:	3:	Reps:
4:	Reps:	4:	Reps:
5:	Reps:	5:	Reps:

FOOD

Breakfast:

Lunch:

Dinner:

Snacks: Crap: Booze:

LIFE

Caring, connecting, committing:

How did you do?   ☐ Amazing   ☐ Not Bad   ☐ Shameful

Plans for tomorrow:

Friday ☐ ☐ ☐

How was your night?

Morning mood: Resting Heart Rate:

EXERCISE

CARDIO

Time and/or distance: Level: Heart Rate Max: Recovery:

STRENGTH: UPPER BODY & BACK		STRENGTH: LEGS & ABS	
1:	Reps:	1:	Reps:
2:	Reps:	2:	Reps:
3:	Reps:	3:	Reps:
4:	Reps:	4:	Reps:
5:	Reps:	5:	Reps:

FOOD

Breakfast:

Lunch:

Dinner:

Snacks: Crap: Booze:

LIFE

Caring, connecting, committing:

How did you do?   ☐ Amazing   ☐ Not Bad   ☐ Shameful

Plans for tomorrow:

Saturday __|__|__|

How was your night?

Morning mood: _____ Resting Heart Rate: _____

E X E R C I S E

CARDIO

Time and/or distance: _____ Level: _____ Heart Rate Max: _____ Recovery: _____

STRENGTH: UPPER BODY & BACK		STRENGTH: LEGS & ABS	
1:	Reps:	1:	Reps:
2:	Reps:	2:	Reps:
3:	Reps:	3:	Reps:
4:	Reps:	4:	Reps:
5:	Reps:	5:	Reps:

F O O D

Breakfast:

Lunch:

Dinner:

Snacks: _____ Crap: _____ Booze: _____

L I F E

Caring, connecting, committing:

How did you do? ☐ Amazing ☐ Not Bad ☐ Shameful

Plans for tomorrow:

Sunday __|__|__|

How was your night?

Morning mood: _____ Resting Heart Rate: _____

E X E R C I S E

CARDIO

Time and/or distance: _____ Level: _____ Heart Rate Max: _____ Recovery: _____

STRENGTH: UPPER BODY & BACK		STRENGTH: LEGS & ABS	
1:	Reps:	1:	Reps:
2:	Reps:	2:	Reps:
3:	Reps:	3:	Reps:
4:	Reps:	4:	Reps:
5:	Reps:	5:	Reps:

F O O D

Breakfast:

Lunch:

Dinner:

Snacks: _____ Crap: _____ Booze: _____

L I F E

Caring, connecting, committing:

How did you do? ☐ Amazing ☐ Not Bad ☐ Shameful

Plans for tomorrow:

44 week

Exercise & Diet Plan for the Week

	MONDAY	TUESDAY	WEDNESDAY	THURSDAY	FRIDAY	SATURDAY	SUNDAY
CARDIO							
WEIGHTS							

Weight at beginning of week: Weight at end of week:

Goals for the week:

Ideas for caring, connecting, committing:

CHRIS SAYS: DEFAULT TO YES

When someone asks you to do something, to join into some activity, say yes.
It's easy—especially for men—to say, "Naw, the hell with it." Well, don't.
Solitude can actually kill you. So, work at developing new friends. And hang
on to the old ones. It'll keep you alive.

Monday ⎵ | | |

How was your night?

Morning mood: Resting Heart Rate:

E X E R C I S E

CARDIO

Time and/or distance: Level: Heart Rate Max: Recovery:

STRENGTH: UPPER BODY & BACK		STRENGTH: LEGS & ABS	
1:	Reps:	1:	Reps:
2:	Reps:	2:	Reps:
3:	Reps:	3:	Reps:
4:	Reps:	4:	Reps:
5:	Reps:	5:	Reps:

F O O D

Breakfast:

Lunch:

Dinner:

Snacks: Crap: Booze:

L I F E

Caring, connecting, committing:

How did you do?   ☐ Amazing   ☐ Not Bad   ☐ Shameful

Plans for tomorrow:

Tuesday ___|__|__

How was your night?

Morning mood: Resting Heart Rate:

EXERCISE

CARDIO

Time and/or distance: Level: Heart Rate Max: Recovery:

STRENGTH: UPPER BODY & BACK		STRENGTH: LEGS & ABS	
1:	Reps:	1:	Reps:
2:	Reps:	2:	Reps:
3:	Reps:	3:	Reps:
4:	Reps:	4:	Reps:
5:	Reps:	5:	Reps:

FOOD

Breakfast:

Lunch:

Dinner:

Snacks: Crap: Booze:

LIFE

Caring, connecting, committing:

How did you do? ☐ Amazing ☐ Not Bad ☐ Shameful

Plans for tomorrow:

Wednesday ___|__|__

How was your night?

Morning mood: Resting Heart Rate:

EXERCISE

CARDIO

Time and/or distance: Level: Heart Rate Max: Recovery:

STRENGTH: UPPER BODY & BACK		STRENGTH: LEGS & ABS	
1:	Reps:	1:	Reps:
2:	Reps:	2:	Reps:
3:	Reps:	3:	Reps:
4:	Reps:	4:	Reps:
5:	Reps:	5:	Reps:

FOOD

Breakfast:

Lunch:

Dinner:

Snacks: Crap: Booze:

LIFE

Caring, connecting, committing:

How did you do? ☐ Amazing ☐ Not Bad ☐ Shameful

Plans for tomorrow:

Thursday␣␣| |

How was your night?

Morning mood:␣␣␣␣␣␣Resting Heart Rate:

EXERCISE

CARDIO

Time and/or distance:␣␣␣␣Level:␣␣␣␣Heart Rate Max:␣␣␣␣Recovery:

STRENGTH: UPPER BODY & BACK		STRENGTH: LEGS & ABS	
1:	Reps:	1:	Reps:
2:	Reps:	2:	Reps:
3:	Reps:	3:	Reps:
4:	Reps:	4:	Reps:
5:	Reps:	5:	Reps:

FOOD

Breakfast:

Lunch:

Dinner:

Snacks:␣␣␣␣Crap:␣␣␣␣Booze:

LIFE

Caring, connecting, committing:

How did you do?␣␣☐ Amazing␣␣☐ Not Bad␣␣☐ Shameful

Plans for tomorrow:

Friday␣␣| |

How was your night?

Morning mood:␣␣␣␣␣␣Resting Heart Rate:

EXERCISE

CARDIO

Time and/or distance:␣␣␣␣Level:␣␣␣␣Heart Rate Max:␣␣␣␣Recovery:

STRENGTH: UPPER BODY & BACK		STRENGTH: LEGS & ABS	
1:	Reps:	1:	Reps:
2:	Reps:	2:	Reps:
3:	Reps:	3:	Reps:
4:	Reps:	4:	Reps:
5:	Reps:	5:	Reps:

FOOD

Breakfast:

Lunch:

Dinner:

Snacks:␣␣␣␣Crap:␣␣␣␣Booze:

LIFE

Caring, connecting, committing:

How did you do?␣␣☐ Amazing␣␣☐ Not Bad␣␣☐ Shameful

Plans for tomorrow:

Saturday ⎸ ⎸ ⎸

How was your night?

Morning mood: Resting Heart Rate:

EXERCISE

CARDIO

Time and/or distance: Level: Heart Rate Max: Recovery:

STRENGTH: UPPER BODY & BACK		STRENGTH: LEGS & ABS	
1:	Reps:	1:	Reps:
2:	Reps:	2:	Reps:
3:	Reps:	3:	Reps:
4:	Reps:	4:	Reps:
5:	Reps:	5:	Reps:

FOOD

Breakfast:

Lunch:

Dinner:

Snacks: Crap: Booze:

LIFE

Caring, connecting, committing:

How did you do? ☐ Amazing ☐ Not Bad ☐ Shameful

Plans for tomorrow:

Sunday ⎸ ⎸ ⎸

How was your night?

Morning mood: Resting Heart Rate:

EXERCISE

CARDIO

Time and/or distance: Level: Heart Rate Max: Recovery:

STRENGTH: UPPER BODY & BACK		STRENGTH: LEGS & ABS	
1:	Reps:	1:	Reps:
2:	Reps:	2:	Reps:
3:	Reps:	3:	Reps:
4:	Reps:	4:	Reps:
5:	Reps:	5:	Reps:

FOOD

Breakfast:

Lunch:

Dinner:

Snacks: Crap: Booze:

LIFE

Caring, connecting, committing:

How did you do? ☐ Amazing ☐ Not Bad ☐ Shameful

Plans for tomorrow:

45 week

Exercise & Diet Plan for the Week

	MONDAY	TUESDAY	WEDNESDAY	THURSDAY	FRIDAY	SATURDAY	SUNDAY
CARDIO							
WEIGHTS							

Weight at beginning of week: Weight at end of week:

Goals for the week:

Ideas for caring, connecting, committing:

HARRY SAYS: REMEMBER COLIN POWELL

No surprise: People who work hard to keep up their connections to others—and who maintain full and meaningful lives themselves—are more optimistic. But what's not so obvious is that people who simply *decide* to approach life with an optimistic attitude actually create their own luck and good feeling. Colin Powell was right: Relentless optimism is a force multiplier.

Monday ___ ___ ___

How was your night?

Morning mood: Resting Heart Rate:

EXERCISE

CARDIO

Time and/or distance: Level: Heart Rate Max: Recovery:

STRENGTH: UPPER BODY & BACK		**STRENGTH: LEGS & ABS**	
1:	Reps:	1:	Reps:
2:	Reps:	2:	Reps:
3:	Reps:	3:	Reps:
4:	Reps:	4:	Reps:
5:	Reps:	5:	Reps:

FOOD

Breakfast:

Lunch:

Dinner:

Snacks: Crap: Booze:

LIFE

Caring, connecting, committing:

How did you do? ☐ Amazing ☐ Not Bad ☐ Shameful

Plans for tomorrow:

Tuesday ___ | | |

How was your night?

Morning mood: Resting Heart Rate:

E X E R C I S E

CARDIO

Time and/or distance: Level: Heart Rate Max: Recovery:

STRENGTH: UPPER BODY & BACK		STRENGTH: LEGS & ABS	
1:	Reps:	1:	Reps:
2:	Reps:	2:	Reps:
3:	Reps:	3:	Reps:
4:	Reps:	4:	Reps:
5:	Reps:	5:	Reps:

F O O D

Breakfast:

Lunch:

Dinner:

Snacks: Crap: Booze:

L I F E

Caring, connecting, committing:

How did you do?   ☐ Amazing   ☐ Not Bad   ☐ Shameful

Plans for tomorrow:

Wednesday ___ | | |

How was your night?

Morning mood: Resting Heart Rate:

E X E R C I S E

CARDIO

Time and/or distance: Level: Heart Rate Max: Recovery:

STRENGTH: UPPER BODY & BACK		STRENGTH: LEGS & ABS	
1:	Reps:	1:	Reps:
2:	Reps:	2:	Reps:
3:	Reps:	3:	Reps:
4:	Reps:	4:	Reps:
5:	Reps:	5:	Reps:

F O O D

Breakfast:

Lunch:

Dinner:

Snacks: Crap: Booze:

L I F E

Caring, connecting, committing:

How did you do?   ☐ Amazing   ☐ Not Bad   ☐ Shameful

Plans for tomorrow:

Thursday | | |

How was your night?

Morning mood: Resting Heart Rate:

E X E R C I S E

CARDIO

Time and/or distance: Level: Heart Rate Max: Recovery:

STRENGTH: UPPER BODY & BACK		STRENGTH: LEGS & ABS	
1:	Reps:	1:	Reps:
2:	Reps:	2:	Reps:
3:	Reps:	3:	Reps:
4:	Reps:	4:	Reps:
5:	Reps:	5:	Reps:

F O O D

Breakfast:

Lunch:

Dinner:

Snacks: Crap: Booze:

L I F E

Caring, connecting, committing:

How did you do?   ☐ Amazing ☐ Not Bad ☐ Shameful

Plans for tomorrow:

Friday | | |

How was your night?

Morning mood: Resting Heart Rate:

E X E R C I S E

CARDIO

Time and/or distance: Level: Heart Rate Max: Recovery:

STRENGTH: UPPER BODY & BACK		STRENGTH: LEGS & ABS	
1:	Reps:	1:	Reps:
2:	Reps:	2:	Reps:
3:	Reps:	3:	Reps:
4:	Reps:	4:	Reps:
5:	Reps:	5:	Reps:

F O O D

Breakfast:

Lunch:

Dinner:

Snacks: Crap: Booze:

L I F E

Caring, connecting, committing:

How did you do?   ☐ Amazing ☐ Not Bad ☐ Shameful

Plans for tomorrow:

Saturday___|__|__|

How was your night?

Morning mood: Resting Heart Rate:

E X E R C I S E

CARDIO

Time and/or distance:	Level:	Heart Rate Max:	Recovery:

STRENGTH: UPPER BODY & BACK		STRENGTH: LEGS & ABS	
1:	Reps:	1:	Reps:
2:	Reps:	2:	Reps:
3:	Reps:	3:	Reps:
4:	Reps:	4:	Reps:
5:	Reps:	5:	Reps:

F O O D

Breakfast:

Lunch:

Dinner:

Snacks:	Crap:	Booze:

L I F E

Caring, connecting, committing:

How did you do? ☐ Amazing ☐ Not Bad ☐ Shameful

Plans for tomorrow:

Sunday___|__|__|

How was your night?

Morning mood: Resting Heart Rate:

E X E R C I S E

CARDIO

Time and/or distance:	Level:	Heart Rate Max:	Recovery:

STRENGTH: UPPER BODY & BACK		STRENGTH: LEGS & ABS	
1:	Reps:	1:	Reps:
2:	Reps:	2:	Reps:
3:	Reps:	3:	Reps:
4:	Reps:	4:	Reps:
5:	Reps:	5:	Reps:

F O O D

Breakfast:

Lunch:

Dinner:

Snacks:	Crap:	Booze:

L I F E

Caring, connecting, committing:

How did you do? ☐ Amazing ☐ Not Bad ☐ Shameful

Plans for tomorrow:

Exercise & Diet Plan for the Week

	MONDAY	TUESDAY	WEDNESDAY	THURSDAY	FRIDAY	SATURDAY	SUNDAY
CARDIO							
WEIGHTS							

Weight at beginning of week: Weight at end of week:

Goals for the week:

Ideas for caring, connecting, committing:

CHRIS SAYS: THINK ABOUT YOUR RESTING METABOLISM

When you exercise, you don't burn all that many calories—maybe 300 to 400 calories during an hour-long workout. Nice, but not huge. What *is* huge is that when you build up your aerobic base, your body burns far more calories when it is resting than it used to. So changing your *resting metabolism* is what leads to serious weight loss. Think of that the next time you're complaining about the treadmill.

Monday ___ ___ ___

How was your night?

Morning mood: Resting Heart Rate:

EXERCISE

CARDIO

Time and/or distance: Level: Heart Rate Max: Recovery:

STRENGTH: UPPER BODY & BACK		STRENGTH: LEGS & ABS	
1:	Reps:	1:	Reps:
2:	Reps:	2:	Reps:
3:	Reps:	3:	Reps:
4:	Reps:	4:	Reps:
5:	Reps:	5:	Reps:

FOOD

Breakfast:

Lunch:

Dinner:

Snacks: Crap: Booze:

LIFE

Caring, connecting, committing:

How did you do? ☐ Amazing ☐ Not Bad ☐ Shameful

Plans for tomorrow:

Tuesday _ | | |_

How was your night?

Morning mood: Resting Heart Rate:

E X E R C I S E

CARDIO

Time and/or distance: Level: Heart Rate Max: Recovery:

STRENGTH: UPPER BODY & BACK		STRENGTH: LEGS & ABS	
1:	Reps:	1:	Reps:
2:	Reps:	2:	Reps:
3:	Reps:	3:	Reps:
4:	Reps:	4:	Reps:
5:	Reps:	5:	Reps:

F O O D

Breakfast:

Lunch:

Dinner:

Snacks: Crap: Booze:

L I F E

Caring, connecting, committing:

How did you do?   ☐ Amazing ☐ Not Bad ☐ Shameful

Plans for tomorrow:

Wednesday _ | | |_

How was your night?

Morning mood: Resting Heart Rate:

E X E R C I S E

CARDIO

Time and/or distance: Level: Heart Rate Max: Recovery:

STRENGTH: UPPER BODY & BACK		STRENGTH: LEGS & ABS	
1:	Reps:	1:	Reps:
2:	Reps:	2:	Reps:
3:	Reps:	3:	Reps:
4:	Reps:	4:	Reps:
5:	Reps:	5:	Reps:

F O O D

Breakfast:

Lunch:

Dinner:

Snacks: Crap: Booze:

L I F E

Caring, connecting, committing:

How did you do?   ☐ Amazing ☐ Not Bad ☐ Shameful

Plans for tomorrow:

Thursday | | |

How was your night?

Morning mood: Resting Heart Rate:

E X E R C I S E

CARDIO

Time and/or distance: Level: Heart Rate Max: Recovery:

STRENGTH: UPPER BODY & BACK		STRENGTH: LEGS & ABS	
1:	Reps:	1:	Reps:
2:	Reps:	2:	Reps:
3:	Reps:	3:	Reps:
4:	Reps:	4:	Reps:
5:	Reps:	5:	Reps:

F O O D

Breakfast:

Lunch:

Dinner:

Snacks: Crap: Booze:

L I F E

Caring, connecting, committing:

How did you do?   ☐ Amazing ☐ Not Bad ☐ Shameful

Plans for tomorrow:

Friday | | |

How was your night?

Morning mood: Resting Heart Rate:

E X E R C I S E

CARDIO

Time and/or distance: Level: Heart Rate Max: Recovery:

STRENGTH: UPPER BODY & BACK		STRENGTH: LEGS & ABS	
1:	Reps:	1:	Reps:
2:	Reps:	2:	Reps:
3:	Reps:	3:	Reps:
4:	Reps:	4:	Reps:
5:	Reps:	5:	Reps:

F O O D

Breakfast:

Lunch:

Dinner:

Snacks: Crap: Booze:

L I F E

Caring, connecting, committing:

How did you do?   ☐ Amazing ☐ Not Bad ☐ Shameful

Plans for tomorrow:

Saturday _ | | |

How was your night?

Morning mood: Resting Heart Rate:

E X E R C I S E

CARDIO

Time and/or distance: Level: Heart Rate Max: Recovery:

STRENGTH: UPPER BODY & BACK		STRENGTH: LEGS & ABS	
1:	Reps:	1:	Reps:
2:	Reps:	2:	Reps:
3:	Reps:	3:	Reps:
4:	Reps:	4:	Reps:
5:	Reps:	5:	Reps:

F O O D

Breakfast:

Lunch:

Dinner:

Snacks: Crap: Booze:

L I F E

Caring, connecting, committing.

How did you do?   ☐ Amazing   ☐ Not Bad   ☐ Shameful

Plans for tomorrow:

Sunday _ | | |

How was your night?

Morning mood: Resting Heart Rate:

E X E R C I S E

CARDIO

Time and/or distance: Level: Heart Rate Max: Recovery:

STRENGTH: UPPER BODY & BACK		STRENGTH: LEGS & ABS	
1:	Reps:	1:	Reps:
2:	Reps:	2:	Reps:
3:	Reps:	3:	Reps:
4:	Reps:	4:	Reps:
5: ,	Reps:	5:	Reps:

F O O D

Breakfast:

Lunch:

Dinner:

Snacks: Crap: Booze:

L I F E

Caring, connecting, committing:

How did you do?   ☐ Amazing   ☐ Not Bad   ☐ Shameful

Plans for tomorrow:

Exercise & Diet Plan for the Week

	MONDAY	TUESDAY	WEDNESDAY	THURSDAY	FRIDAY	SATURDAY	SUNDAY
CARDIO							
WEIGHTS							

Weight at beginning of week: Weight at end of week:

Goals for the week:

Ideas for caring, connecting, committing:

HARRY SAYS: GET THE RIGHT BIKE FOR YOU

Biking is just about the ideal aerobic sport. It's great for you, it's low impact and safe for your knees, and you can do it until you are very old. If you haven't biked for a while, you may want to get what some call a "comfort" or "hybrid" bike which will allow you to sit upright. They are less expensive, easier to ride, and a good way to reintroduce yourself to the sport.

Monday __ __ __

How was your night?

Morning mood: Resting Heart Rate:

E X E R C I S E

CARDIO

Time and/or distance: Level: Heart Rate Max: Recovery:

STRENGTH: UPPER BODY & BACK		STRENGTH: LEGS & ABS	
1:	Reps:	1:	Reps:
2:	Reps:	2:	Reps:
3:	Reps:	3:	Reps:
4:	Reps:	4:	Reps:
5:	Reps:	5:	Reps:

F O O D

Breakfast:

Lunch:

Dinner:

Snacks: Crap: Booze:

L I F E

Caring, connecting, committing:

How did you do? ☐ Amazing ☐ Not Bad ☐ Shameful

Plans for tomorrow:

Tuesday_____

How was your night?

Morning mood:　　　　　　Resting Heart Rate:

EXERCISE

CARDIO

Time and/or distance:　　　Level:　　　Heart Rate Max:　　　Recovery:

STRENGTH: UPPER BODY & BACK		STRENGTH: LEGS & ABS	
1:	Reps:	1:	Reps:
2:	Reps:	2:	Reps:
3:	Reps:	3:	Reps:
4:	Reps:	4:	Reps:
5:	Reps:	5:	Reps:

FOOD

Breakfast:

Lunch:

Dinner:

Snacks:　　　　　　　　　Crap:　　　　　　　Booze:

LIFE

Caring, connecting, committing:

How did you do?　☐ Amazing　☐ Not Bad　☐ Shameful

Plans for tomorrow.

Wednesday_____

How was your night?

Morning mood:　　　　　　Resting Heart Rate:

EXERCISE

CARDIO

Time and/or distance:　　　Level:　　　Heart Rate Max:　　　Recovery:

STRENGTH: UPPER BODY & BACK		STRENGTH: LEGS & ABS	
1:	Reps:	1:	Reps:
2:	Reps:	2:	Reps:
3:	Reps:	3:	Reps:
4:	Reps:	4:	Reps:
5:	Reps:	5:	Reps:

FOOD

Breakfast:

Lunch:

Dinner:

Snacks:　　　　　　　　　Crap:　　　　　　　Booze:

LIFE

Caring, connecting, committing:

How did you do?　☐ Amazing　☐ Not Bad　☐ Shameful

Plans for tomorrow:

Thursday ⌐⌐ ⌐

How was your night?

Morning mood: Resting Heart Rate:

CARDIO

Time and/or distance: Level: Heart Rate Max: Recovery:

STRENGTH: UPPER BODY & BACK		STRENGTH: LEGS & ABS	
1:	Reps:	1:	Reps:
2:	Reps:	2:	Reps:
3:	Reps:	3:	Reps:
4:	Reps:	4:	Reps:
5:	Reps:	5:	Reps:

Breakfast:

Lunch:

Dinner:

Snacks: Crap: Booze:

Caring, connecting, committing:

How did you do? ☐ Amazing ☐ Not Bad ☐ Shameful

Plans for tomorrow:

Friday ⌐⌐ ⌐

How was your night?

Morning mood: Resting Heart Rate:

CARDIO

Time and/or distance: Level: Heart Rate Max: Recovery:

STRENGTH: UPPER BODY & BACK		STRENGTH: LEGS & ABS	
1:	Reps:	1:	Reps:
2:	Reps:	2:	Reps:
3:	Reps:	3:	Reps:
4:	Reps:	4:	Reps:
5:	Reps:	5:	Reps:

Breakfast:

Lunch:

Dinner:

Snacks: Crap: Booze:

Caring, connecting, committing:

How did you do? ☐ Amazing ☐ Not Bad ☐ Shameful

Plans for tomorrow:

Saturday _____ | | |

How was your night?

Morning mood: Resting Heart Rate:

EXERCISE

CARDIO

Time and/or distance: Level: Heart Rate Max: Recovery:

STRENGTH: UPPER BODY & BACK		STRENGTH: LEGS & ABS	
1:	Reps:	1:	Reps:
2:	Reps:	2:	Reps:
3:	Reps:	3:	Reps:
4:	Reps:	4:	Reps:
5:	Reps:	5:	Reps:

FOOD

Breakfast:

Lunch:

Dinner:

Snacks: Crap: Booze:

LIFE

Caring, connecting, committing:

How did you do? ☐ Amazing ☐ Not Bad ☐ Shameful

Plans for tomorrow:

Sunday _____ | | |

How was your night?

Morning mood: Resting Heart Rate:

EXERCISE

CARDIO

Time and/or distance: Level: Heart Rate Max: Recovery:

STRENGTH: UPPER BODY & BACK		STRENGTH: LEGS & ABS	
1:	Reps:	1:	Reps:
2:	Reps:	2:	Reps:
3:	Reps:	3:	Reps:
4:	Reps:	4:	Reps:
5:	Reps:	5:	Reps:

FOOD

Breakfast:

Lunch:

Dinner:

Snacks: Crap: Booze:

LIFE

Caring, connecting, committing:

How did you do? ☐ Amazing ☐ Not Bad ☐ Shameful

Plans for tomorrow:

Exercise & Diet Plan for the Week

	MONDAY	TUESDAY	WEDNESDAY	THURSDAY	FRIDAY	SATURDAY	SUNDAY
CARDIO							
WEIGHTS							

Weight at beginning of week: _____ Weight at end of week: _____

Goals for the week: _____

Ideas for caring, connecting, committing: _____

_____

CHRIS SAYS: GET A GREAT ROAD BIKE AS SOON AS YOU CAN

Harry's right about biking, but so many people just dog it in biking and never get the full benefit of the sport. Wear your heart rate monitor and go hard enough to get your heart rate up to at least 60% of your max. And—listen up!—buy yourself a decent bike as soon as you can. Get into the sport and then take advantage of the amazing developments in equipment that have taken place over the last decade or so. A great bike is a great motivator.

Monday _____ | | |

How was your night? _____

Morning mood: _____ Resting Heart Rate: _____

EXERCISE

CARDIO

Time and/or distance: _____ Level: _____ Heart Rate Max: _____ Recovery: _____

STRENGTH: UPPER BODY & BACK		STRENGTH: LEGS & ABS	
1:	Reps:	1:	Reps:
2:	Reps:	2:	Reps:
3:	Reps:	3:	Reps:
4:	Reps:	4:	Reps:
5:	Reps:	5:	Reps:

FOOD

Breakfast:

Lunch:

Dinner:

Snacks: _____ Crap: _____ Booze: _____

LIFE

Caring, connecting, committing:

How did you do? ☐ Amazing ☐ Not Bad ☐ Shameful

Plans for tomorrow:

Tuesday ___ | | |

How was your night?

Morning mood: Resting Heart Rate:

E X E R C I S E

CARDIO

Time and/or distance: Level: Heart Rate Max: Recovery:

STRENGTH: UPPER BODY & BACK		**STRENGTH: LEGS & ABS**	
1:	Reps:	1:	Reps:
2:	Reps:	2:	Reps:
3:	Reps:	3:	Reps:
4:	Reps:	4:	Reps:
5:	Reps:	5:	Reps:

F O O D

Breakfast:

Lunch:

Dinner:

Snacks: Crap: Booze:

L I F E

Caring, connecting, committing:

How did you do?   ☐ Amazing   ☐ Not Bad   ☐ Shameful

Plans for tomorrow:

Wednesday ___ | | |

How was your night?

Morning mood: Resting Heart Rate:

E X E R C I S E

CARDIO

Time and/or distance: Level: Heart Rate Max: Recovery:

STRENGTH: UPPER BODY & BACK		**STRENGTH: LEGS & ABS**	
1:	Reps:	1:	Reps:
2:	Reps:	2:	Reps:
3:	Reps:	3:	Reps:
4:	Reps:	4:	Reps:
5:	Reps:	5:	Reps:

F O O D

Breakfast:

Lunch:

Dinner:

Snacks: Crap: Booze:

L I F E

Caring, connecting, committing:

How did you do?   ☐ Amazing   ☐ Not Bad   ☐ Shameful

Plans for tomorrow:

Thursday _|_|_|_

How was your night?

Morning mood: Resting Heart Rate:

EXERCISE

CARDIO

Time and/or distance: Level: Heart Rate Max: Recovery:

STRENGTH: UPPER BODY & BACK		STRENGTH: LEGS & ABS	
1:	Reps:	1:	Reps:
2:	Reps:	2:	Reps:
3:	Reps:	3:	Reps:
4:	Reps:	4:	Reps:
5:	Reps:	5:	Reps:

FOOD

Breakfast:

Lunch:

Dinner:

Snacks: Crap: Booze:

LIFE

Caring, connecting, committing:

How did you do?   ☐ Amazing   ☐ Not Bad   ☐ Shameful

Plans for tomorrow:

Friday _|_|_|_

How was your night?

Morning mood: Resting Heart Rate:

EXERCISE

CARDIO

Time and/or distance: Level: Heart Rate Max: Recovery:

STRENGTH: UPPER BODY & BACK		STRENGTH: LEGS & ABS	
1: .	Reps:	1:	Reps:
2:	Reps:	2:	Reps:
3:	Reps:	3:	Reps:
4:	Reps:	4:	Reps:
5:	Reps:	5:	Reps:

FOOD

Breakfast:

Lunch:

Dinner:

Snacks: Crap: Booze:

LIFE

Caring, connecting, committing:

How did you do?   ☐ Amazing   ☐ Not Bad   ☐ Shameful

Plans for tomorrow:

Saturday␣␣␣|␣|␣|

How was your night?
Morning mood: Resting Heart Rate:

EXERCISE

CARDIO

Time and/or distance: Level: Heart Rate Max: Recovery:

STRENGTH: UPPER BODY & BACK		STRENGTH: LEGS & ABS	
1:	Reps:	1:	Reps:
2:	Reps:	2:	Reps:
3:	Reps:	3:	Reps:
4:	Reps:	4:	Reps:
5:	Reps:	5:	Reps:

FOOD

Breakfast:

Lunch:

Dinner:

Snacks: Crap: Booze:

LIFE

Caring, connecting, committing:

How did you do?   ☐ Amazing   ☐ Not Bad   ☐ Shameful

Plans for tomorrow:

Sunday␣␣␣|␣|␣|

How was your night?
Morning mood: Resting Heart Rate:

EXERCISE

CARDIO

Time and/or distance: Level: Heart Rate Max: Recovery:

STRENGTH: UPPER BODY & BACK		STRENGTH: LEGS & ABS	
1:	Reps:	1:	Reps:
2:	Reps:	2:	Reps:
3:	Reps:	3:	Reps:
4:	Reps:	4:	Reps:
5:	Reps:	5:	Reps:

FOOD

Breakfast:

Lunch:

Dinner:

Snacks: Crap: Booze:

LIFE

Caring, connecting, committing:

How did you do?   ☐ Amazing   ☐ Not Bad   ☐ Shameful

Plans for tomorrow:

Exercise & Diet Plan for the Week

	MONDAY	TUESDAY	WEDNESDAY	THURSDAY	FRIDAY	SATURDAY	SUNDAY
CARDIO							
WEIGHTS							

Weight at beginning of week: _____ Weight at end of week: _____

Goals for the week: _____

Ideas for caring, connecting, committing: _____

CHRIS SAYS: DON'T WHINE

Whine about your spouse. Whine about your selfish, rotten children. Whine about your job. But not about your workouts. Your workout is your sacred friend and must be treated accordingly. So stop complaining. We're saving lives here, for heaven's sake!

Monday ___ ___ ___

How was your night?

Morning mood: _____ Resting Heart Rate: _____

EXERCISE

CARDIO

Time and/or distance: _____ Level: _____ Heart Rate Max: _____ Recovery: _____

STRENGTH: UPPER BODY & BACK		STRENGTH: LEGS & ABS	
1:	Reps:	1:	Reps:
2:	Reps:	2:	Reps:
3:	Reps:	3:	Reps:
4:	Reps:	4:	Reps:
5:	Reps:	5:	Reps:

FOOD

Breakfast:

Lunch:

Dinner:

Snacks: _____ Crap: _____ Booze: _____

LIFE

Caring, connecting, committing:

How did you do? ☐ Amazing ☐ Not Bad ☐ Shameful

Plans for tomorrow:

Tuesday___|___|___|

How was your night?	
Morning mood:	Resting Heart Rate:

E X E R C I S E

CARDIO

Time and/or distance: Level: Heart Rate Max: Recovery:

STRENGTH: UPPER BODY & BACK		STRENGTH: LEGS & ABS	
1:	Reps:	1:	Reps:
2:	Reps:	2:	Reps:
3:	Reps:	3:	Reps:
4:	Reps:	4:	Reps:
5:	Reps:	5:	Reps:

F O O D

Breakfast:

Lunch:

Dinner:

Snacks: Crap: Booze:

L I F E

Caring, connecting, committing:

How did you do?   ☐ Amazing ☐ Not Bad ☐ Shameful

Plans for tomorrow:

Wednesday___|___|___|

How was your night?	
Morning mood:	Resting Heart Rate:

E X E R C I S E

CARDIO

Time and/or distance: Level: Heart Rate Max: Recovery:

STRENGTH: UPPER BODY & BACK		STRENGTH: LEGS & ABS	
1:	Reps:	1:	Reps:
2:	Reps:	2:	Reps:
3:	Reps:	3:	Reps:
4:	Reps:	4:	Reps:
5:	Reps:	5:	Reps:

F O O D

Breakfast:

Lunch:

Dinner:

Snacks: Crap: Booze:

L I F E

Caring, connecting, committing:

How did you do?   ☐ Amazing ☐ Not Bad ☐ Shameful

Plans for tomorrow:

Thursday␣␣|␣|␣|

How was your night?

Morning mood:␣␣␣␣␣Resting Heart Rate:

EXERCISE

CARDIO

Time and/or distance:␣␣␣␣␣Level:␣␣␣␣␣Heart Rate Max:␣␣␣␣␣Recovery:

STRENGTH: UPPER BODY & BACK		STRENGTH: LEGS & ABS	
1:	Reps:	1:	Reps:
2:	Reps:	2:	Reps:
3:	Reps:	3:	Reps:
4:	Reps:	4:	Reps:
5:	Reps:	5:	Reps:

FOOD

Breakfast:

Lunch:

Dinner:

Snacks:␣␣␣␣␣Crap:␣␣␣␣␣Booze:

LIFE

Caring, connecting, committing:

How did you do?␣␣☐ Amazing␣␣☐ Not Bad␣␣☐ Shameful

Plans for tomorrow:

Friday␣␣|␣|␣|

How was your night?

Morning mood:␣␣␣␣␣Resting Heart Rate:

EXERCISE

CARDIO

Time and/or distance:␣␣␣␣␣Level:␣␣␣␣␣Heart Rate Max:␣␣␣␣␣Recovery:

STRENGTH: UPPER BODY & BACK		STRENGTH: LEGS & ABS	
1:	Reps:	1:	Reps:
2:	Reps:	2:	Reps:
3:	Reps:	3:	Reps:
4:	Reps:	4:	Reps:
5:	Reps:	5:	Reps:

FOOD

Breakfast:

Lunch:

Dinner:

Snacks:␣␣␣␣␣Crap:␣␣␣␣␣Booze:

LIFE

Caring, connecting, committing:

How did you do?␣␣☐ Amazing␣␣☐ Not Bad␣␣☐ Shameful

Plans for tomorrow:

Saturday___|___|___|

How was your night?	
Morning mood:	Resting Heart Rate:

E X E R C I S E

CARDIO

Time and/or distance:	Level:	Heart Rate Max:	Recovery:

STRENGTH: UPPER BODY & BACK		STRENGTH: LEGS & ABS	
1:	Reps:	1:	Reps:
2:	Reps:	2:	Reps:
3:	Reps:	3:	Reps:
4:	Reps:	4:	Reps:
5:	Reps:	5:	Reps:

F O O D

Breakfast:

Lunch:

Dinner:

Snacks:	Crap:	Booze:

L I F E

Caring, connecting, committing:

How did you do? ☐ Amazing ☐ Not Bad ☐ Shameful

Plans for tomorrow:

Sunday___|___|___|

How was your night?	
Morning mood:	Resting Heart Rate:

E X E R C I S E

CARDIO

Time and/or distance:	Level:	Heart Rate Max:	Recovery:

STRENGTH: UPPER BODY & BACK		STRENGTH: LEGS & ABS	
1:	Reps:	1:	Reps:
2:	Reps:	2:	Reps:
3:	Reps:	3:	Reps:
4:	Reps:	4:	Reps:
5:	Reps:	5:	Reps:

F O O D

Breakfast:

Lunch:

Dinner:

Snacks:	Crap:	Booze:

L I F E

Caring, connecting, committing:

How did you do? ☐ Amazing ☐ Not Bad ☐ Shameful

Plans for tomorrow:

Exercise & Diet Plan for the Week

	MONDAY	TUESDAY	WEDNESDAY	THURSDAY	FRIDAY	SATURDAY	SUNDAY
CARDIO							
WEIGHTS							

Weight at beginning of week: Weight at end of week:

Goals for the week:

Ideas for caring, connecting, committing:

CHRIS SAYS: **DON'T *WINE* EITHER, OR NOT MUCH**

One of the bits of bad luck that comes with aging is that we are less able to handle spirits. There are population studies that suggest that small amounts of wine or liquor are good for you, but those amounts are very small, especially as you age. Two glasses of wine a day are plenty for men, and one is the limit for women. More than that can lead to very serious problems. So, don't forget to count.

Monday | | |

How was your night?

Morning mood: Resting Heart Rate:

E X E R C I S E

CARDIO

Time and/or distance: Level: Heart Rate Max: Recovery:

STRENGTH: UPPER BODY & BACK		**STRENGTH: LEGS & ABS**	
1:	Reps:	1:	Reps:
2:	Reps:	2:	Reps:
3:	Reps:	3:	Reps:
4:	Reps:	4:	Reps:
5:	Reps:	5:	Reps:

F O O D

Breakfast:

Lunch:

Dinner:

Snacks: Crap: Booze:

L I F E

Caring, connecting, committing:

How did you do?   ☐ Amazing   ☐ Not Bad   ☐ Shameful

Plans for tomorrow:

Tuesday ___ | | |

How was your night?

Morning mood: Resting Heart Rate:

EXERCISE

CARDIO

Time and/or distance: Level: Heart Rate Max: Recovery:

STRENGTH: UPPER BODY & BACK		STRENGTH: LEGS & ABS	
1:	Reps:	1:	Reps:
2:	Reps:	2:	Reps:
3:	Reps:	3:	Reps:
4:	Reps:	4:	Reps:
5:	Reps:	5:	Reps:

FOOD

Breakfast:

Lunch:

Dinner:

Snacks: Crap: Booze:

LIFE

Caring, connecting, committing:

How did you do? ☐ Amazing ☐ Not Bad ☐ Shameful

Plans for tomorrow:

Wednesday ___ | | |

How was your night?

Morning mood: Resting Heart Rate:

EXERCISE

CARDIO

Time and/or distance: Level: Heart Rate Max: Recovery:

STRENGTH: UPPER BODY & BACK		STRENGTH: LEGS & ABS	
1:	Reps:	1:	Reps:
2:	Reps:	2:	Reps:
3:	Reps:	3:	Reps:
4:	Reps:	4:	Reps:
5:	Reps:	5:	Reps:

FOOD

Breakfast:

Lunch:

Dinner:

Snacks: Crap: Booze:

LIFE

Caring, connecting, committing:

How did you do? ☐ Amazing ☐ Not Bad ☐ Shameful

Plans for tomorrow:

Thursday ⎸ ⎸ ⎸

How was your night?

Morning mood: Resting Heart Rate:

EXERCISE

CARDIO

Time and/or distance: Level: Heart Rate Max: Recovery:

STRENGTH: UPPER BODY & BACK		STRENGTH: LEGS & ABS	
1:	Reps:	1:	Reps:
2:	Reps:	2:	Reps:
3:	Reps:	3:	Reps:
4:	Reps:	4:	Reps:
5:	Reps:	5:	Reps:

FOOD

Breakfast:

Lunch:

Dinner:

Snacks: Crap: Booze:

LIFE

Caring, connecting, committing:

How did you do?   ☐ Amazing   ☐ Not Bad   ☐ Shameful

Plans for tomorrow:

Friday ⎸ ⎸ ⎸

How was your night?

Morning mood: Resting Heart Rate:

EXERCISE

CARDIO

Time and/or distance: Level: Heart Rate Max: Recovery:

STRENGTH: UPPER BODY & BACK		STRENGTH: LEGS & ABS	
1:	Reps:	1:	Reps:
2:	Reps:	2:	Reps:
3:	Reps:	3:	Reps:
4:	Reps:	4:	Reps:
5:	Reps:	5:	Reps:

FOOD

Breakfast:

Lunch:

Dinner:

Snacks: Crap: Booze:

LIFE

Caring, connecting, committing:

How did you do?   ☐ Amazing   ☐ Not Bad   ☐ Shameful

Plans for tomorrow:

Saturday ▢ ▢ ▢

How was your night?

Morning mood: Resting Heart Rate:

EXERCISE

CARDIO

Time and/or distance: Level: Heart Rate Max: Recovery:

STRENGTH: UPPER BODY & BACK		STRENGTH: LEGS & ABS	
1:	Reps:	1:	Reps:
2:	Reps:	2:	Reps:
3:	Reps:	3:	Reps:
4:	Reps:	4:	Reps:
5:	Reps:	5:	Reps:

FOOD

Breakfast:

Lunch:

Dinner:

Snacks: Crap: Booze:

LIFE

Caring, connecting, committing:

How did you do?   ☐ Amazing ☐ Not Bad ☐ Shameful

Plans for tomorrow:

Sunday ▢ ▢ ▢

How was your night?

Morning mood: Resting Heart Rate:

EXERCISE

CARDIO

Time and/or distance: Level: Heart Rate Max: Recovery:

STRENGTH: UPPER BODY & BACK		STRENGTH: LEGS & ABS	
1:	Reps:	1:	Reps:
2:	Reps:	2:	Reps:
3:	Reps:	3:	Reps:
4:	Reps:	4:	Reps:
5:	Reps:	5:	Reps:

FOOD

Breakfast:

Lunch:

Dinner:

Snacks: Crap: Booze:

LIFE

Caring, connecting, committing:

How did you do?   ☐ Amazing ☐ Not Bad ☐ Shameful

Plans for tomorrow:

Exercise & Diet Plan for the Week

	MONDAY	TUESDAY	WEDNESDAY	THURSDAY	FRIDAY	SATURDAY	SUNDAY
CARDIO							
WEIGHTS							

Weight at beginning of week: _____ Weight at end of week: _____

Goals for the week: _____

Ideas for caring, connecting, committing: _____

CHRIS SAYS: OKAY, LISTEN TO HARRY THIS TIME

Sad to say, Harry's quite right about the dear old spirits. I am constantly reminded—because I am so slow to learn—that I can handle much less these days. Drink too much wine and . . . the next day I feel OLD! I've gone to too much trouble to be functionally younger to take those chances. Oh, you know, I risk it once in a while, just for fun. I do fun, Harry does virtue, but this time he's right.

Monday ___ | | |

How was your night? _____

Morning mood: _____ Resting Heart Rate: _____

EXERCISE

CARDIO

Time and/or distance: _____ Level: _____ Heart Rate Max: _____ Recovery: _____

STRENGTH: UPPER BODY & BACK		STRENGTH: LEGS & ABS	
1:	Reps:	1:	Reps:
2:	Reps:	2:	Reps:
3:	Reps:	3:	Reps:
4:	Reps:	4:	Reps:
5:	Reps:	5:	Reps:

FOOD

Breakfast:

Lunch:

Dinner:

Snacks: _____ Crap: _____ Booze: _____

LIFE

Caring, connecting, committing:

How did you do? ☐ Amazing ☐ Not Bad ☐ Shameful

Plans for tomorrow:

Tuesday_ | | |

How was your night?	
Morning mood:	Resting Heart Rate:

EXERCISE

CARDIO

Time and/or distance:	Level:	Heart Rate Max:	Recovery:

STRENGTH: UPPER BODY & BACK		STRENGTH: LEGS & ABS	
1:	Reps:	1:	Reps:
2:	Reps:	2:	Reps:
3:	Reps:	3:	Reps:
4:	Reps:	4:	Reps:
5:	Reps:	5:	Reps:

FOOD

Breakfast:

Lunch:

Dinner:

Snacks:	Crap:	Booze:

LIFE

Caring, connecting, committing:

How did you do? ☐ Amazing ☐ Not Bad ☐ Shameful

Plans for tomorrow:

Wednesday_ | | |

How was your night?	
Morning mood:	Resting Heart Rate:

EXERCISE

CARDIO

Time and/or distance:	Level:	Heart Rate Max:	Recovery:

STRENGTH: UPPER BODY & BACK		STRENGTH: LEGS & ABS	
1:	Reps:	1:	Reps:
2:	Reps:	2:	Reps:
3:	Reps:	3:	Reps:
4:	Reps:	4:	Reps:
5:	Reps:	5:	Reps:

FOOD

Breakfast:

Lunch:

Dinner:

Snacks:	Crap:	Booze:

LIFE

Caring, connecting, committing:

How did you do? ☐ Amazing ☐ Not Bad ☐ Shameful

Plans for tomorrow:

Thursday ___ | | |

How was your night?

Morning mood: Resting Heart Rate:

E X E R C I S E

CARDIO

Time and/or distance: Level: Heart Rate Max: Recovery:

STRENGTH: UPPER BODY & BACK		STRENGTH: LEGS & ABS	
1:	Reps:	1:	Reps:
2:	Reps:	2:	Reps:
3:	Reps:	3:	Reps:
4:	Reps:	4:	Reps:
5:	Reps:	5:	Reps:

F O O D

Breakfast:

Lunch:

Dinner:

Snacks: Crap: Booze:

L I F E

Caring, connecting, committing:

How did you do?   ☐ Amazing   ☐ Not Bad   ☐ Shameful

Plans for tomorrow:

Friday ___ | | |

How was your night?

Morning mood: Resting Heart Rate:

E X E R C I S E

CARDIO

Time and/or distance: Level: Heart Rate Max: Recovery:

STRENGTH: UPPER BODY & BACK		STRENGTH: LEGS & ABS	
1:	Reps:	1:	Reps:
2:	Reps:	2:	Reps:
3:	Reps:	3:	Reps:
4:	Reps:	4:	Reps:
5:	Reps:	5:	Reps:

F O O D

Breakfast:

Lunch:

Dinner:

Snacks: Crap: Booze:

L I F E

Caring, connecting, committing:

How did you do?   ☐ Amazing   ☐ Not Bad   ☐ Shameful

Plans for tomorrow:

Saturday ___|___|___

How was your night?	
Morning mood:	Resting Heart Rate:

EXERCISE

CARDIO

Time and/or distance: Level: Heart Rate Max: Recovery:

STRENGTH: UPPER BODY & BACK		STRENGTH: LEGS & ABS	
1:	Reps:	1:	Reps:
2:	Reps:	2:	Reps:
3:	Reps:	3:	Reps:
4:	Reps:	4:	Reps:
5:	Reps:	5:	Reps:

FOOD

Breakfast:

Lunch:

Dinner:

Snacks: Crap: Booze:

LIFE

Caring, connecting, committing:

How did you do?   ☐ Amazing   ☐ Not Bad   ☐ Shameful

Plans for tomorrow:

Sunday ___|___|___

How was your night?	
Morning mood:	Resting Heart Rate:

EXERCISE

CARDIO

Time and/or distance: Level: Heart Rate Max: Recovery:

STRENGTH: UPPER BODY & BACK		STRENGTH: LEGS & ABS	
1:	Reps:	1:	Reps:
2:	Reps:	2:	Reps:
3:	Reps:	3:	Reps:
4:	Reps:	4:	Reps:
5:	Reps:	5:	Reps:

FOOD

Breakfast:

Lunch:

Dinner:

Snacks: Crap: Booze:

LIFE

Caring, connecting, committing:

How did you do?   ☐ Amazing   ☐ Not Bad   ☐ Shameful

Plans for tomorrow:

Exercise & Diet Plan for the Week

	MONDAY	TUESDAY	WEDNESDAY	THURSDAY	FRIDAY	SATURDAY	SUNDAY
CARDIO							
WEIGHTS							

Weight at beginning of week: _____ Weight at end of week: _____

Goals for the week: _____

Ideas for caring, connecting, committing: _____

HARRY SAYS: CONNECT AND COMMIT

Almost as important as physical exercise is connecting with and committing to other people. Isolation is a grave peril, and it can age you a lot. Make a conscious effort to work and play with your fellow creatures. It sends a strong message to your body to be younger. And who doesn't want that?

Oh, by the way, now that you've made it through a year of exercise, celebrate your accomplishments with your friends. But don't forget to keep going back to the gym tomorrow . . . and tomorrow . . . and . . .

Monday ___

How was your night?

Morning mood: _____ Resting Heart Rate: _____

EXERCISE

CARDIO

Time and/or distance: _____ Level: _____ Heart Rate Max: _____ Recovery: _____

STRENGTH: UPPER BODY & BACK		STRENGTH: LEGS & ABS	
1:	Reps:	1:	Reps:
2:	Reps:	2:	Reps:
3:	Reps:	3:	Reps:
4:	Reps:	4:	Reps:
5:	Reps:	5:	Reps:

FOOD

Breakfast:

Lunch:

Dinner:

Snacks: _____ Crap: _____ Booze: _____

LIFE

Caring, connecting, committing:

How did you do? ☐ Amazing ☐ Not Bad ☐ Shameful

Plans for tomorrow:

Tuesday__|_|__|

How was your night?

Morning mood:　　　　　　Resting Heart Rate:

EXERCISE

CARDIO

Time and/or distance:　　　　Level:　　　Heart Rate Max:　　Recovery:

STRENGTH: UPPER BODY & BACK		STRENGTH: LEGS & ABS	
1:	Reps:	1:	Reps:
2:	Reps:	2:	Reps:
3:	Reps:	3:	Reps:
4:	Reps:	4:	Reps:
5:	Reps:	5:	Reps:

FOOD

Breakfast:

Lunch:

Dinner:

Snacks:　　　　　　　　　Crap:　　　　　　Booze:

LIFE

Caring, connecting, committing:

How did you do?　☐Amazing　☐Not Bad　☐Shameful

Plans for tomorrow:

Wednesday__|_|__|

How was your night?

Morning mood:　　　　　　Resting Heart Rate:

EXERCISE

CARDIO

Time and/or distance:　　　　Level:　　　Heart Rate Max:　　Recovery:

STRENGTH: UPPER BODY & BACK		STRENGTH: LEGS & ABS	
1:	Reps:	1:	Reps:
2:	Reps:	2:	Reps:
3:	Reps:	3:	Reps:
4:	Reps:	4:	Reps:
5:	Reps:	5:	Reps:

FOOD

Breakfast:

Lunch:

Dinner:

Snacks:　　　　　　　　　Crap:　　　　　　Booze:

LIFE

Caring, connecting, committing:

How did you do?　☐Amazing　☐Not Bad　☐Shameful

Plans for tomorrow:

Thursday | | |

How was your night?

Morning mood: Resting Heart Rate:

EXERCISE

CARDIO

Time and/or distance: Level: Heart Rate Max: Recovery:

STRENGTH: UPPER BODY & BACK		STRENGTH: LEGS & ABS	
1:	Reps:	1:	Reps:
2:	Reps:	2:	Reps:
3:	Reps:	3:	Reps:
4:	Reps:	4:	Reps:
5:	Reps:	5:	Reps:

FOOD

Breakfast:

Lunch:

Dinner:

Snacks: Crap: Booze:

LIFE

Caring, connecting, committing:

How did you do? ☐ Amazing ☐ Not Bad ☐ Shameful

Plans for tomorrow:

Friday | | |

How was your night?

Morning mood: Resting Heart Rate:

EXERCISE

CARDIO

Time and/or distance: Level: Heart Rate Max: Recovery:

STRENGTH: UPPER BODY & BACK		STRENGTH: LEGS & ABS	
1:	Reps:	1:	Reps:
2:	Reps:	2:	Reps:
3:	Reps:	3:	Reps:
4:	Reps:	4:	Reps:
5:	Reps:	5:	Reps:

FOOD

Breakfast:

Lunch:

Dinner:

Snacks: Crap: Booze:

LIFE

Caring, connecting, committing:

How did you do? ☐ Amazing ☐ Not Bad ☐ Shameful

Plans for tomorrow:

Saturday ___ | ___ | ___

How was your night?

Morning mood: Resting Heart Rate:

EXERCISE

CARDIO

Time and/or distance: Level: Heart Rate Max: Recovery:

STRENGTH: UPPER BODY & BACK		STRENGTH: LEGS & ABS	
1:	Reps:	1:	Reps:
2:	Reps:	2:	Reps:
3:	Reps:	3:	Reps:
4:	Reps:	4:	Reps:
5:	Reps:	5:	Reps:

FOOD

Breakfast:

Lunch:

Dinner:

Snacks: Crap: Booze:

LIFE

Caring, connecting, committing:

How did you do? ☐ Amazing ☐ Not Bad ☐ Shameful

Plans for tomorrow:

Sunday ___ | ___ | ___

How was your night?

Morning mood: Resting Heart Rate:

EXERCISE

CARDIO

Time and/or distance: Level: Heart Rate Max: Recovery:

STRENGTH: UPPER BODY & BACK		STRENGTH: LEGS & ABS	
1:	Reps:	1:	Reps:
2:	Reps:	2:	Reps:
3:	Reps:	3:	Reps:
4:	Reps:	4:	Reps:
5:	Reps:	5:	Reps:

FOOD

Breakfast:

Lunch:

Dinner:

Snacks: Crap: Booze:

LIFE

Caring, connecting, committing:

How did you do? ☐ Amazing ☐ Not Bad ☐ Shameful

Plans for tomorrow:

MY STATS AT THE END OF THE YEAR

My weight: _____

My waking heart rate: _____

My recovery rate: _____

My true maximum heart rate: _____

My blood pressure: _____

My cholesterol: _____

My normal aerobic activity (how many minutes spent on an elliptical machine, road bike, etc.): _____

How many days a week: _____

My normal weight activity (how much weight you lift, or what machines you use): _____

Frequency of normal weight activity (how many days a week): _____

MY GOALS FOR NEXT YEAR

1. _____

_____

_____

2. _____

_____

_____

3. _____

_____

_____

4. _____

_____

_____

5. _____

_____

_____

6. _____

_____

_____

7. _____

_____

_____

NOTES:

NOTES:

NOTES:

NOTES:

About the Authors

Chris Crowley and Henry S. Lodge, M.D., are the authors of *Younger Next Year* and *Younger Next Year for Women*. They are also patient and doctor, and the enthusiastic creators of the Younger Next Year™ program. A graduate of Harvard and the University of Virginia Law School, Mr. Crowley was, until his retirement in 1990, a litigator and partner at Davis Polk & Wardwell in Manhattan. He is married to the portraitist Hilary Cooper. Dr. Lodge, who graduated from the University of Pennsylvania and Columbia University Medical School, is a board-certified internist in New York City. The head of a 23-doctor practice, he is a member of the clinical faculty at Columbia University's College of Physicians and Surgeons.

BY THE SAME AUTHORS

NOW IN PAPERBACK, the *New York Times* bestselling book for men that heralded a paradigm shift in our view of aging. Drawing on the latest scientific findings, *Younger Next Year* teaches men how they can become *functionally younger every year*—and continue living like fifty-year-olds well into their eighties.

NOW IN PAPERBACK, the bestselling program that teaches women how to turn back their biological clocks and live healthier, more active lives into their eighties and beyond. *Younger Next Year for Women* covers everything from osteoporosis to sexuality to finances, and is packed with simple—but powerful— motivational rules designed to fit women's lifestyles.